Second Medical Opinion

Sergio A. Chacón M.

Published by Sergio A. Chacón M., 2023.

While every precaution has been taken in the preparation of this book, the publisher assumes no responsibility for errors or omissions, or for damages resulting from the use of the information contained herein.

SECOND MEDICAL OPINION

First edition. November 10, 2023.

ISBN: 979-8215691762

Written by Sergio A. Chacón M..

About Dr. Sergio A. Chacon M.

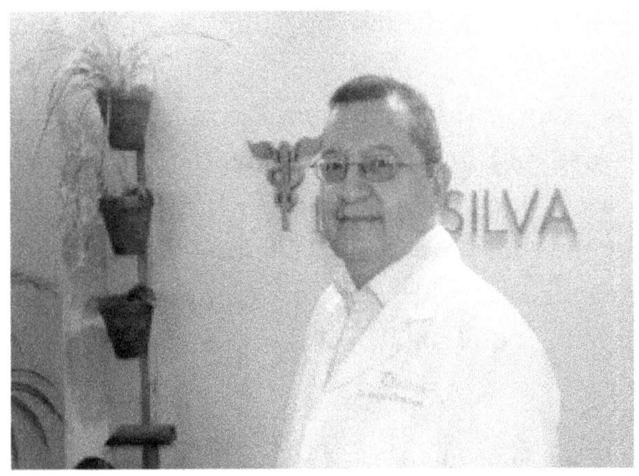

Venezuelan doctor graduated in 1986 from the University of Los Andes and practiced Conventional Medicine exclusively for 15 years. He worked in more than 10 health institutions in different cities in Venezuela and traveled the long road from rural medicine and rotating internship to internal medicine residency and then cardiology.

In 1999, being the District Cardiologist of the western axis of the Carabobo State based at the Bejuma Hospital and feeling highly disappointed by the ineffectiveness of conventional medicine to heal heart patients, he decided to venture into the paths of other medicine starting with Naturopathy.

After seeing better results in his patients when applying natural treatments, he decided to delve deeper into this field and moved to the US to train in Phytotherapy, Nutrition and Holistic Iridology.

In 2008 he managed to homologate his medical degree in Spain and settled in Las Palmas de Gran Canaria, where he founded a 3-year Naturopathy program for professionals from different fields and coordinated it for 10 years, achieving several promotions of Naturopaths.

In 2016 he founded the first Integrative Medicine Center in Las Palmas de Gran Canaria incorporating the services of Medicine, Naturopathy, Acupuncture, Nutrition, Psychology and Physiotherapy, and was the Medical Director of said center until February 2020.

In the last 3 years he has dedicated himself to private medical consultation, the completion of new master's degrees, such as the one in Microbiota taken with the Regenera group of Barcelona, Spain, in 2022, the production of online courses and editing books, this being his first book.

Dedication

To the memory of my parents, to whom I owe everything I am, because they not only gave me life, but also each one of the principles that have allowed me to get to where I have gotten, even to the point of sitting down to write this book, which now sees the light and I can offer to you.

To my beloved wife and life partner, with whom I shared my medical training and we have lived together a long history of 37 years of professional experience, and to whom I owe the encouragement and concern to explore the paths of other medicine and thus discover many truths that have allowed me to free myself from the fundamentalist slavery of conventional hospital medicine.

To my two daughters, who have always been a source of inspiration to continue moving forward in the search for a better world for them and in that search, I have found unexpected and revealing paths.

To Ramón Plasencia, who taught me the value of doing things correctly, to Ana Merchan Mujica, who taught me the immense value that the study and understanding of history has in the future of people, to Juan T. González of whom I learned the importance of discipline and methodology in the study of medicine, from Gustavo Arriechi, who made me see that he who only knows medicine, not even medicine knows, from Keshava Baht, my teacher of tropical naturism.

To Germán Alberti for his teaching of naturopathy, to David Pesek, for his passion and dedication to holistic iridology and to each one of the professors and teachers who have passed through my student life and who contributed to carve and model in me the professional that I am today.

To every one of the people who have visited my medical consultation, because thanks to their experience as patients and their trust, I have been able to know the thousand faces of the disease and assess the effectiveness of both conventional and non-conventional medicine, and thus understanding the true nature of Integrative Medicine.

Note to Readers

This book is based on bibliographic research and the author's personal experience. It is offered to the public with the understanding that it is not intended as a medical or other consultation for the individual reader. No one should use the information contained in the work as a substitute for the advice of a licensed medical professional, and the reader should consult with his or her licensed primary care physician before using any of the remedies, supplements, plants, medications, and the like described in this book. The Author disclaims any type of responsibility in relation to any loss, injury, or damage, caused directly or indirectly by the use of this book.

Foreword

The book you hold in your hands is full of life. First, because it contains the story of a piece of the life of 14 people who visited my medical office in search of a solution for their terrible health problem, which seemed incurable, which had made them wander through multiple offices of various specialists and try various treatments, without achieving a stable improvement and much less achieving total healing, thus being immersed in a life of very poor quality and marked by the suffering and hopelessness of a disease that seemed invincible.

Second, because you will be able to read my medical arguments and the paths that I took to help those 14 people achieve the cure of their diseases, applying the best of both medicines, conventional and unconventional. You will also be able to receive directly from my lips each one of the messages that I wish to transmit to you to offer you an alternative, hope and light. in the tunnel of darkness in which you or one of your most loved ones may find yourself, suffering the rigors of an illness that does not want to leave you and that your doctors have not been able to eradicate.

I have titled the introduction "The other side of Medicine", and there you will find a detailed description, without being as extensive as it could be, of both conventional medicine and non-conventional medicine, so that you know the origin and the evolution that both have had in the course of history and you can understand the reason why in the present day of the 21st century it seems that in the Western Hemisphere there are two medicines, different and confronting.

Conventional medicine is what dominates all scenarios, what reigns in all hospitals, what rules in all international health institutions and what governs the destiny of the vast majority of patients who seek medical assistance to alleviate their ailments and of the vast majority of doctors who dedicate their lives to the care of these patients, turning the former into happy slaves to pharmacies and their illnesses and the latter into the pawns of a highly lucrative market which works every time. They write a medical prescription, thinking and believing that they are doing the best for their patients, while remaining hypnotized and enchanted under the yoke of pseudoscientific slavery of the powerful chemical pharmaceutical industry.

While the other medicine, the non-conventional one, baptized as Traditional by the World Health Organization (WHO), has been growing since its resurgence in the sixties of the 20th century, taking on an increasingly careful and scientific character. convincing and seeking integration to give way to the birth of Integrative Medicine, which uses all types of treatment, with a scientific basis to offer patients the best possible results in the resolution of their disease.

The rest of the book is made up of 14 chapters and in each of them you will find a real story, of real people, who, being patients, are in search of a resolution to their diseases, chronic, degenerative and often described as incurable by their treating doctors grew tired of feeling frustrated and disappointed in a medicine that only offered them medications, laboratory tests and special examinations, and the much vaunted claim of control of their symptoms, but without offering the desired promise of definitive healing.

To embark on the adventure of searching for a different alternative, in the fields of other medicine, undergoing little-known processes and treatments, assuming the responsibility of fighting and working for their recovery and handing over their last hopes in the hands of a medicine criticized and disqualified by the official media, but glorified and recommended by friends and family who tried it and were healed.

I invite you to visit Pablo in chapter 1, so that you can learn about his story marked by a genetic disease that affected his heart and at 45 years old they did not give him more than 3 to 5 years to live, and they were evaluating him to see if they included him on a list for a heart transplant.

In chapter 2 you will find Ruth, a 57-year-old teacher who suddenly began to suffer from red, painful, burning spots that appeared on her extremities and then took over the trunk and went alone to the 3 or 4 days and they forced her to rest at home so as not to expose the ugly appearance they gave her.

You can see Teresa in chapter 3, a 46-year-old woman who suffered and cried every time it was time to eat, because almost everything she ate was bad for her and caused very uncomfortable digestive discomfort, gas, intestinal bloating, reflux, heartburn, colic, cramps and even diarrhea. Teresa had been suffering from this ordeal for 6 years and none of the specialists she had visited gave her a solution.

Pedro is in chapter 4, a 26-year-old young man, who was surprised and scared by a condition of erectile dysfunction and intense physical fatigue that was causing him problems with his partner, and he was even more surprised after the doctors told him that he was suffering of hypothyroidism and had to take a hormone-based medication for the rest of his life.

Luisa awaits you in chapter 5, a pretty 29-year-old girl who had gotten married at the age of 27 and had been trying to get pregnant for 2 years without success and who had resorted to an assisted fertility clinic and after having invested time and money in a long and expensive treatment, with all the hope of becoming a mother, ended in failure that plunged her into deep sadness.

María, a 43-year-old woman, awaits you in chapter 6 to tell you about the terrible scare she experienced with some vomiting of blood that she had on a Sunday night, which warranted her transfer to the emergency room, where fortunately they managed to stabilize her with blood transfusions. However, her scare was greater when, after performing tests, the doctors referred her to hematology to rule out Leukemia.

In chapter 7 you can visit Ramón, a 46-year-old man who worked in front of the public at a school and who suddenly suffered from severe facial paralysis and after having been seen, first in the medical emergency room and three days later, for his GP, he did not receive any kind of treatment and was only given an appointment to see an ENT specialist and a Physiotherapist, 45 days later.

In chapter 8 you will be able to find out how Felipe, a 51-year-old man, was taken to the emergency room on the night of December 27 with the diagnosis of acute appendicitis, and that when he was opened in the surgical ward, they found a malignant tumor. 7cm in the right colon, with 2 positive lymph nodes and liver involvement.

Esteban is a 15-year-old young man who awaits you in chapter 9 and will share with you the struggle he faced with a diagnosis of attention deficit hyperactivity disorder (ADHD).

And with the battle that it represented to abandon the psychiatric medication that he had been taking for a few years, which was causing serious side effects.

In chapter 10 you will be surprised by the case of Yadira, a 36-year-old woman who was very close to losing her life due to anorexia nervosa that she suffered for almost a year, which surprisingly went unnoticed by all the doctors who treated her at that time, those who classified her as having fibromyalgia, multiple chemical sensitivity and made her spend a lot of money with expensive medical tests and treatments that were unsuccessful.

Luis, a 36-year-old gardener is in chapter 11, he is going to tell you how he became asthmatic without ever having been allergic, and how he entered a spiral of flu, pharyngitis and repetitive pneumonia, which took him to the pulmonology office and try several treatments without any improvement.

You can visit the young Silvia, barely 12 years old, in chapter 12. This girl will tell you how she was diagnosed with a disease called *Juvenile Rheumatoid Arthritis*, after several fingers on both hands became swollen. She was treated with a very strong medication called methotrexate, which was not curing her arthritis and to top it all off, it was causing damage to her kidneys.

Juana will be waiting for you in chapter 13, she is a 31-year-old nurse who was temporarily unable to work due to chronic low back pain that did not allow her to lead a normal life and was being monitored by neurosurgery for a possible spinal surgery that she didn't want to.

You will finally meet Victor in chapter 14, a 45-year-old police officer who was suffering from chronic dizziness and after some tests they detected an arrhythmia in his heart with a very slow rhythm and the possibility of requiring a pacemaker.

My intention is to rescue a lesson from each of the experiences lived by these people, both from their frustration and disappointment at not having received a satisfactory solution from their conventional doctors, and from the surprise and novelty of having achieved a spectacular improvement in their quality of life and the total and definitive healing of most of the illnesses suffered by them, after having sought a second opinion in the field of other medicine.

I invite you with all my heart to accompany me on this journey full of experiences, anguish, tears, and joys, emanating from the lives of people who were confronted with health problems that were difficult to solve and who with their bravery and courage decided to take a step forward. against the current to discover the world of so-called Integrative Medicine, where a gratifying and surprise awaited them that would lead them back to a life full of health.

Finally, I give you an epilogue with my final reflections, which I have personalized for four groups of readers. I start with **healthy readers**, those privileged people who have never been sick or are not sick now, but are people concerned about staying in a state of well-being. Then I address the people who, at the time of reading this book, suffer from some illness, they are the *sick patients*, who are probably reading this book in search of an alternative to their chronic illness. The third group of readers are *medical students*, the replacement generation, and future doctors, in whose hands will be the type of medicine we will have in the coming decades.

The fourth and last group of readers are *doctors*, those who, strangely and unexpectedly, have read this book, and have learned through its pages, that there is another medicine, which is also very broad and solid, and although different in its methods, it could offer great benefits to patients, where conventional treatments have failed.

Introduction

The other side of Medicine

We can define Conventional Medicine as the system by which doctors and other health professionals, such as nurses, pharmacists, and therapists, treat symptoms and diseases through medications, radiation, or surgery. This form of medicine is also called biomedicine, allopathic medicine, mainstream medicine, western medicine, or orthodox medicine.

Conventional Medicine represents the dominant form of medicine in the Western Hemisphere, while in the Eastern Hemisphere, the medical scene is fundamentally occupied by the so-called Traditional Medicine, with Traditional Chinese Medicine and Indian Ayurvedic Medicine being very representative. In the Eastern Hemisphere, Conventional Medicine occupies a secondary place.

Conventional Medicine is about 150 years old, and we must look for its foundations in the middle of the 19th century, the so-called golden century of knowledge and science. In the second half of that century, some discoveries occurred that laid the foundations for this form of medicine, the most important being the following:

In 1848 Claude Bernard, the great physiologist of that century and official founder of experimental medicine, discovered the first enzyme, pancreatic lipase. In that year, ether began to be used to sedate patients before surgery.

The medical figure par excellence of this period was Rudolf Virchow. He developed the disciplines of hygiene and social medicine, at the origins of current preventive medicine. It is the same Virchow who postulated the theory of "Omnia cell to cell" (every cell comes from another cell) and explained living organisms as structures made up of cells. Shortly before his death, in 1902, he was a candidate for the Nobel Prize in Physiology and Medicine, along with the Spanish Santiago Ramón y Cajal, who would finally obtain the award in 1906.

Louis Pasteur, although he did not study medicine, can be considered one of the most influential researchers in the history of 19th century medicine. His training as a chemist led him to design a method for observing chemical substances using polarized light, which opened the doors to the study of microorganisms, demonstrating that in fermentation processes, phenomena of "spontaneous generation" were not produced, but of proliferation of previously present microorganisms.

Joseph Lister would later apply this knowledge by developing the surgical practice of asepsis and antisepsis using heat, thus managing to drastically reduce mortality rates after operations, the main obstacle to the definitive takeoff of surgery. The definitive blow to infectious diseases (after vaccines and asepsis) was dealt by Alexander Fleming at the beginning of the 20th century with the discovery of penicillin, the first antibiotic.

On November 8, 1895, Wilhelm Rontgen, a German physicist, managed to produce a new type of electromagnetic radiation at the wavelengths corresponding to those currently called X-rays. For this discovery he would receive the Nobel Prize in Physics in 1901.

It is the first of the diagnostic imaging techniques that will allow us to observe the inside of the human body in vivo. In 1896, physicists Henri Becquerel, Pierre Curie and Marie Curie discovered radioactivity, which would give rise to Nuclear Medicine.

Between the 19th and 20th centuries, three medical conceptions or paradigms developed, all of them heirs of the scientific model, mainly biological and with philosophical foundations in positivism:

1.-Anatomoclinical Paradigm: the origin of the disease is in the injury.

2.-Physiopathological Paradigm: the origin is sought in the altered processes.

3.-Etiological Paradigm: the origin may lie in external causes.

Among the most outstanding doctors of this 20th century, it is worth highlighting Sigmund Freud, the great revolutionary of psychiatry, Robert Koch, discoverer of the bacillus that causes tuberculosis, Paul Ehrlich, father of immunology, Harvey Cushing, father of neurosurgery, or Alexander Fleming, discoverer of penicillin, which began the "antibiotic era" of medicine.

In 1948, the World Health Organization (WHO) was founded under the protection of the United Nations (UN), the first international medical organization specialized in managing health prevention, promotion, and intervention policies worldwide.

In 1978, the Alma-Ata International Conference on Primary Health Care was held, where the declaration of the bio-psycho-social concept of health was revealed.

As well as the crucial importance of social measures (adequate supply of drinking water and food, vaccinations...) and primary health care to improve the health level of the populations. The motto (finally not fulfilled) of this conference was Health for all in the year 2000.

Technical medicine, capable of unraveling the secrets of the human body through devices such as Magnetic Resonance, has generated a "medicalizing" social current, in which problems and behaviors become diseases. In this way, two objectives are achieved: transferring responsibility from the individual to the "disease" and leaving its solution in the hands of technology.

However, parallel to this evidence, the development of pharmacology at an industrial and economic level has made 20th century medicine dependent on medicine as an icon of health. Aspirin, synthesized by Félix Hoffmann in 1897, has become one of the symbols of the culture of that century. These contradictory features, a dehumanized and commercialized medicine, but which has managed to eradicate diseases such as smallpox or poliomyelitis and which has managed to increase average life expectancy above 70 years in most developed countries, are the synthesis of conventional modern medicine.

In the last decades of the 20th century, psychiatry developed a psychopharmacological school based on the premise that the mechanism of action of psychotropic drugs revealed in turn the pathophysiological mechanism secondary to the psychic disorder, thus approaching Neurophysiology.

More technical achievements that should be highlighted are blood transfusion, carried out successfully for the first time in this century thanks to the work on blood groups developed by Karl Landsteiner, or organ transplantation, championed, not by the first, but by the most media and successful of its developers, Christian Barnard, the first surgeon to successfully perform a heart transplant.

Molecular genetics was born, and the applications of physics were developed in different areas of medicine: the use of radioisotopes, electrophoresis, chromatography, spectrophotometry, the use of lasers, the electron microscope, ultrasound techniques, computed axial tomography or magnetic resonance imaging.

The automation of calculation through computerized systems has transformed 20th century society. This tool has been a great boost for many applied sciences such as medicine. Possibly the greatest medical achievement of the 20th century is the sequencing of the human genome and although it will still take a few decades to understand and take advantage of this enormous wealth of information, there is no doubt that it will represent a new revolution in the way we approach many diseases, and even, in the way of understanding and defining the human being.

In summary, we can point out that the characteristics that best define Conventional Medicine, considering its evolution over the last 150 years, are the following:

*-It is a biologist: it focuses on the problem of health and disease on the biochemical and biological level of the body, without giving hardly any relevance to other levels such as the mental, emotional, energetic, or spiritual.

*-It is mechanistic: it considers the human body as a machine made up of parts, and disease as a damage to one of its parts that must be repaired, eliminated, or changed, to restore health.

*-It is reductionist: it divides the human body into organs and encourages the specialization and super-specialization of doctors to repair each of those organs in the most efficient way possible.

*-It is dehumanized: it sees the human being as a set of individual organs that work as a team and its function revolves around the repair of those organs, without even caring about the name of the person, their origin, their relationship with the environment, his way of thinking, the emotions he manages, nor his lifestyle.

*-It is focused on the Disease: it worships the disease, who is the protagonist in all outpatient clinics, health centers, clinics and hospitals, where hospitalized sick people lie and are called by the name of their illness, and everything the health personnel who work in them focus their work on all aspects related to the disease.

*-It is anti-health: the word health almost does not exist in the jargon spoken by health personnel, health promotion is nothing more than an empty name on a door plate, preventive medicine is seen as a sterile desert when that no one wants to go, health education is a term that almost no one remembers or knows its meaning. All people who come seeking medical assistance must have some symptom of illness, because if they are completely healthy and only seek to maintain their well-being or avoid illness, they are grotesquely expelled from all medical consultations.

*-It is mercantilist: it places economic values above human values. The important thing is to generate money in large quantities. Each of the diseases and the specialty that treats them have become highly lucrative businesses, true companies.

Like the cancer company, cardiovascular diseases, diabetes, autoimmune diseases, etc., whose pharmacological and surgical treatments are highly lucrative and generate billions of dollars each year.

*-It is experimental: all its therapeutic procedures must be experimented on both animals and humans, to enjoy validation and legal authorization. However, the violation of scientific ethics, deception, and influence peddling are common procedures to obtain the health permits required by official bodies, with the sole objective of launching their new products to keep the pharmacological market in force. and enslaved the patient population by chronically consuming most of the drugs produced for life.

*-It is corporatist: it works like a gigantic corporation that has taken over all the institutions that make up society and the life of each nation. The immense economic wealth it generates, which is infinite, like the stars of the universe, has allowed it to penetrate and control all the mechanisms of social power and no institution has been saved from falling into its networks.

In the 150 years of its existence, it has taken over the universities where doctors are trained and has modified the curriculum or study plans at will and rigorously adapting it to its interests, thus eliminating subjects such as nutrition, botany, and environmental medicine and history of medicine so that doctors are not aware of the origins of medicine and are ignorant in nutrition and phytotherapy; while focusing on pharmacology, biochemistry, anatomy and pathology so that doctors only think and practice based on the dominant medicine paradigm.

In addition to controlling the training of doctors at all the universities in the Western Hemisphere, it also controls the WHO, all the ministries of health of each country, the medical colleges, the specialized media (scientific journals) and non-specialized media (regular press).

Even all political institutions have fallen into their networks, so that each of these sectors only does and says what they are ordered, to guarantee the survival and strengthening of an institution that has parasitized the bowels of humanity, which in its unbridled and excessive desire for power and control, the serious threat of death and self-destruction.

The other side of medicine, which represents the counterpart of modern official medicine, is the so-called Non-Conventional Medicine, which is the daughter and heir of ancestral, hygienist, naturist, environmentalist and vitalist medicine, which believes in an innate *Force of healing* and conceives health as the expression of a harmonious balance between all the bodies that make up the human being, the energetic, mental, emotional, spiritual, biochemical, biological, physiological and social body.

Non-Conventional Medicine has received many names, some of them given by Conventional Medicine itself, many times to mark the differentiation between the two, and other times to disqualify or distort it in the general population. Some of those names are: *"The other Medicine"*, *"Artisanal Medicine"*, *"Alternative Medicine"*, *"Complementary Medicine"*. Other times it has been the same practitioners of Non-Conventional Medicine who have called it different things, to reflect its nature, and in this way, some other names have been tried:

*-**Natural Medicine or Naturopathy:*** refers to the use of natural remedies and methods to recover health and maintain well-being, such as the sun (heliotherapy), water (hydrotherapy), the earth

(geotherapy), etc. It therefore proposes leading a lifestyle attached to the laws of nature to keep us healthy.

*-**Holistic Medicine:** refers to the holistic approach, which means the whole. It is intended to highlight that this form of medicine studies the human being as a totality integrated into a single being, where all their bodies, anatomical, biochemical, mental, energetic, emotional, and spiritual, are interconnected and functioning globally and any imbalance in some of them ends up altering the functioning of the whole. Therefore, its objective is to diagnose possible imbalances in each of the different bodies, to correct them and restore the total health of the organism.

*-**Functional Medicine:** refers to the study of the functionality of each organ and its relationship with all other organs of the body. It aims to evaluate and diagnose disorders or health imbalances that initially affect the function of different organs, causing varied and non-specific symptoms, at a time when there are still no anatomical signs of any injury that can be detected with conventional diagnostic methods, such as radiology, ultrasound, tomography, etc. It bases its diagnoses on the evaluation of biochemical and biomolecular elements that may be altered and are the basis of the functional alteration that is causing the patients' symptoms.

*-**Orthomolecular Medicine:** it is based on the study of the biochemical individuality of each person and on the search for the precise molecular disorder (precision medicine), which may be causing all the disorders that affect the physiology and/or anatomy of the body and that they are responsible for the patient's symptoms.

It states that therapy should be based on the selection of the precise molecules that must be corrected in quantity and quality, at the precise dose, even using mega doses, to correct the biochemical disorder that is at the root of the disease.

*-**Energy Medicine or Bioenergetics:** refers to the set of energies that exist and circulate in our body and that represent the foreground

of the organism's functionality. It speaks of the ***chi*** of Chinese Medicine, which circulates through the meridians that connect all the organs in an intricate network of multiple relationships and connections, or the ***prana*** of Ayurveda, or the luminous, vibrational, electrical, and magnetic energies, electromagnetic, radiofrequency or bioresonance, which are the basis of a wide variety of sophisticated equipment that uses biophysics for the diagnosis and treatment of all alterations of the different energies of our body.

*-**Biological Medicine:*** that which bases its study on the understanding of the functioning of our biology and uses remedies that only exist in living bodies naturally, such as vitamins, minerals, enzymes, trace elements, etc. Therefore, ruling out the use of synthetic and artificial remedies that can be harmful to the body.

*-**Traditional Medicine:*** it is one of the most used terms and the one preferred by the World Health Organization (WHO), to refer to the forms of medicine that are specific to each culture and have an anthropological nature, which has born and has been forged with each type of civilization. It includes *Traditional Naturopathic Medicine, Traditional Chinese Medicine, Ayurvedic Medicine, Indigenous Medicine, Shamanic Medicine,* etc.

At its annual meeting in 2011, the WHO developed a program entitled: "*Strategies 2011 to 2023 to include traditional medicines in national health systems*", thus showing its interest in taking advantage of the benefits of traditional medicines in the resolution of many primary care problems.

The origins of ***Non-Conventional Medicine***, the type of medicine that includes all the names and terms explained in the previous paragraphs, must be sought at the dawn of history, about 5000 years ago, because it was born with the first forms of primitive medicine of the first Western and Eastern civilizations, whose methods have evolved with the history of the different empires and throughout the different eras, such as the Ancient Age, the Middle Ages, the

Renaissance, the Modern Age and the Contemporary Age until reaching the present day .

In the Western Hemisphere the first forms of Traditional Medicine were born with the oldest civilizations, dating back to 4000 years BC, in remote **Mesopotamia and Pharaonic Egypt**, the well-known Persian, Sumerian and Babylonian civilizations flourished. From that stage in history, the first contributions to Medicine were:

.-Medicine had a magical-religious focus, linked to the Gods.

.-They observed the importance of personal and home hygiene to maintain good health

.-They pointed out that inadequate nutrition was the cause of the disease

.-The interrogation of the patient is born, as a basic tool to understand the symptoms.

.-The isolation of the sick and the disposal of excreta were implemented to take care of collective health.

In ancient **Greece**, between 900 and 250 BC, medicine acquired great relevance and momentum, thanks to the figures of great doctors and philosophers.

Who stood out throughout those eight centuries and whose contributions lasted for more than a thousand years. Between the years 900 and 700 BC. The following contributions stood out:

.-Birth of hydrotherapy, thermotherapy, chiromassage and physiotherapy to restore health

.-Empirical knowledge of medicinal plants begins to use them as remedies.

.-The concept of balanced eating and the need for physical exercise to stay healthy arises.

Between the years 700 and 460 BC, the first brilliant figures of medicine emerged in Greece, such as Pythagoras, Alcmaeon, Empedocles and Diogenes of Apollonia, whose contributions to medicine were:

.-The concept of balanced measurement in aspects of health is born

.-The importance of the relationship between nutrition, digestion, fermentation and health was highlighted.

.-The concept of vegetarian food arose for ethics and morals.

.-The theory of humors and the 4 elements (air/earth/fire/water) was born to understand the dynamics of the body.

.-It was proposed that the role of the doctor should be the restoration of the lost balance, in union with nature.

Between the years 450 and 370 BC. The figure and work of who would later be called *Father of Western Medicine* prevailed. Hippocrates, the medical director of Aegean Medicine on the island of Kos, in Greece, developed a form of medicine unique for the time and left a postulate for history, which still exists today. We can summarize the most outstanding aspects of this titanic work as follows.

Hippocrates taught and promulgated that the practice of medicine should be based on several inalienable principles, which were the following:

• Health is the highest of gifts and therefore we must take care of it as our greatest treasure.

• Exercise, professional activity, and social customs are elements that influence health.

• Nature is what heals (*Natura vis Medicatrix*)

• All diseases are curable, however, not all patients are.

• There are Sick and non-Disease: the treatment of each patient must be individualized.

• May your food be your medicine and may your medicine be your food

• The doctor must be an educator, instructor, and facilitator of the healing process.

• When treating the patient, the doctor must try to First do no harm (*Primum Non Nocere*).

- The doctor should always try to find the Root that causes the disease (*Tolle Causam*).

Hippocrates proposed that every disease evolves in three phases, which are as follows:

- The disease appears due to the alteration of raw humors or dirt.
- The reaction of the Physis (body) to dirt generates the symptoms of the disease.
- Healing could occur by improving the processes of elimination of emuntoria and cleansing the humors.

Hippocrates was the first to:

- Associate the climate with health and wrote the first treatise on climatotherapy: "*Of air, water and places*".
- Establish the idea of the *Prognosis* of the disease, when describing its natural evolution.
- Use and encourage fasting, raw fruits and vegetables as detoxifying therapy.
- Use water as a therapeutic agent in hot or cold baths (hydrotherapy).
- Leaving his legacy in a 10-volume collection, the "*Hippocratic Corpus*" that lasted for 1000 years.
- Point out poor diet, intoxication, emotions, and the effect of the weather as causes of illness.
- Write about medical conduct and ethics developing a strict code of behavior based on compassion, commitment, respect, and the doctor's obligation to the patient.
- Collect all his recommendations on professional ethics in the famous "*Hippocratic Oath*".

The last Greek contribution to medicine was given by prominent philosophers between 350 and 250 BC, such as Plato, Socrates, Aristotle, and Erasistratus, who established:

- That the disease was related to a disharmony between the soul and the body.

- The Psychosomatic conception of the disease.
- The importance of verbal Psychotherapy to facilitate the healing of the soul.

Medicine in ancient **Rome** was an extension of Greek medical knowledge. The most notable thing was the creation of several Medical Schools with different approaches, which dominated the medical scene for a certain period. The most notable were the following:

*-Stoic School: Seneca 4 BC. : The most important contributions of this school were the following:

- The idea that illness is punishment for denaturalizing the body with poor health habits.
- We must lead a frugal, simple life, strengthening the body.

*-Ecleptic School, 30 years AD: Celsus and Dioscóride, their most notable contributions were:

- Established 3 forms of therapy: dietetics, herbology and surgery.
- Published the first Materia Medica of Phytotherapy

*-Methodical School, 50 years AD.: Asklepiades and Thesaslio, their contributions were:

- It gave a great boost to hydrotherapy
- Promoted the construction of aqueducts and spas
- Promoted fasting and strict and prolonged diets
- Emphasized the patient's collaboration in healing

*-Pneumatic School, 100 AD.: Galen: It was the most outstanding and his contributions were:

- Developed the *Biological Typology* based on the humors; Phlegmatic, Choleric and Melancholic.
- Developed the approach of treating diseases by their opposites: *Contraria contraris curantur.*
- The medicine (*pharmakon*) could act as medicine or as poison, depending on the use to which it was given.
- Advised the abundant use of medicines: hands of the gods

- The doctor must be a philosopher (*iatros*) and not just a prescriber (*pharmakeüs*)
  - He trusted more in the capacity of reason to treat the sick.
  - He is considered the father of *Rational Therapeutics*.

- His work and his influence extended from the 2nd century to the 18th century.

During the **Middle Ages** (5th to 10th centuries AD), sociopolitical changes occurred that dramatically influenced medicine. Roman medical regulations disappeared, and medical care was controlled by the church.

Many monasteries became healing centers (*Nosocomios*), generating the first concept of hospital. There were many medical practitioners in the town and the urine bottle became the symbol of the doctor. In the 5th century the city of Constantinople became the main center of medical studies and in the 7th century medical knowledge was greatly influenced by ISLAM. The most prominent Arab doctors of the world were: Rhazes 925 AD; prominent physician of Iran, Avicenna 980 AD; the Galen of Islamic culture, Abulcasi 1013 AD, Avenzoar 1148 AD., and Maimonides 1162 AD. The most important contributions of these doctors were:

- Fever was recognized as a defense mechanism of the body against disease.

- The contagious nature of some diseases, such as tuberculosis, was established.

- Cataract surgery and the practice of Tracheostomy began.

In the **Renaissance** period (11th to 18th centuries) some events occurred that gave a great boost to medicine, such as the founding of the first *School of Medicine in Europe in Salerno* (Italy) and in the year 1180 AD. The title of *Doctor of Medicine* was created for the first time.

The Black Death (1347 to 1352) began a period of new interest in research in the field of Medicine. Medicine entered the age of Enlightenment and ushered in a period of remarkable explosion of creative energy, humanistic thought began to replace existing dogmas, and the invention of the printing press helped it spread throughout Europe. Figures such as Leonardo Da Vinci (1452-1519) and Paracelsus (1463-1565) stood out. The most relevant aspects of medicine at that time were:

- A new meaning was given to the medical profession
- Great importance was given to toxins, individual constitution, and psychological conditions
- Anatomy and Alchemy entered a new era of advances.

During the **19th century**, many people still doubted the ability of doctors for not providing solutions to diseases. The high cost of medical services did not allow the working class to attend consultations. It represents the era of patented medicines, all those that bore the name of their inventor. The drugs prepared by doctors, which usually contained toxins such as antimony or mercury, were trusted very little. As a result, interest in herbs was revived. The most prominent medical figures of that time include:

*- Vinzenz Priessnitz, (1799-1851) and Sebastian Kneipp, (1821-1897), : *Fathers of Hydrotherapy.*

.-All diseases have their roots in blood alterations, either because pathogenic substances are present, or because its normal circulation has been disturbed.

.-The disease arose from an unnatural way of living, excess medications, copious meals, strong intellectual or passionate impressions, etc.

.-His therapy was based on eliminating these harmful substances, restoring circulation and invigorating the weakened body, all through water treatment.

.-In their treatments they combined hydropathic practices with diet, outdoor exercises and other recommendations on lifestyle habits.

.-They did not conceive of water as a remedy in itself, but rather the healing agent was the vital force of the sick organism itself.

•.-They believed that: *"The true doctor resides in the human being himself; I only help nature and it cures the disease."*

*-Samuel Hahnemann, (1755-1843) and Constantine Hering (1850): *Fathers of Homeopathy.*

• The word homeopathy derives from the Greek *"homoios"* which means similar and *"pathos"* which means suffering. The same substance that in large doses produces the symptoms of a disease, in minimal doses, cures it.

• The therapeutic action of homeopathic remedies is found in the field of quantum physics.

• The specific electromagnetic frequency of the original substance is recorded in the homeopathic remedy after diluting and shaking. The homeopathic remedy sends the body an *electromagnetic* message that corresponds to the frequency, or pattern, of a disease to stimulate the body's normal healing response.

• Healing progresses from the deepest parts of the body to the extremities, from head to toe and from mental/emotional aspects to physical aspects.

• The healing process begins by eliminating the immediate symptoms and then continues with the old symptoms, which are usually like layers of fever, trauma, or chronic injuries that were treated unsuccessfully or suppressed with conventional medications.

*- Benedict Lust, 1892: *Father of Naturopathy.*

.-Naturopathy was defined as *"a way of life and a healing concept that used different natural means to treat diseases and conditions."*

• Created the term *"natural healing"* which was a combination of North American hygiene, German natural healing, and Kneipp hydrotherapy.

• Is it better to combat diseases with irritating substances, such as vaccines and serums typical of modern superstition, or through harmless forces intrinsic to natural therapeutics, used by this new school of medicine, Naturopathy?

• The Naturopathic Cures Program included: The elimination of bad habits, adopting corrective habits and assuming new principles to live better.

In the **20th century,** in the mid-1930s, Morris Fishbein, editor of the Journal of the American Medical Association (JAMA), embarked on a personal vendetta against naturopathic medicine, which he considered *"quackery."* In that decade the popularity of naturopathy began to decline, due to the introduction of Sulfonamides in the Salk vaccine in 1937, the American public became accustomed to the annual appearance of miracle vaccines and antibiotics.

The craze for technology, the emergence of miracle chemical medicine, interest in surgery, spurred by World War II, the Flexner report, and the death of Benedict Lust in 1945 combined to cause the decline of Natural Medicine or Naturopathic and Natural Healing in the USA.

At the height of their own self-confidence, in the 19th and early 20th centuries, Western doctors attempted to discredit any form of medical treatment other than orthodox.

Despite restrictions and numerous legal actions against unconventional practitioners, Orthodox forces were never able to achieve absolute victory.

Herbal or naturopathic medicine was able to survive and some of it was even adopted as a form of conventional treatment. The same thing happened with other popular therapies such as the famous bone setters, which evolved to become *Chiropractic* and *Osteopathy*. Even some qualified doctors practiced unorthodox techniques, such as hypnosis, homeopathy, manipulative therapies, naturopathy, herbal medicine and eventually acupuncture.

Around 1960, while orthodox medical science had achieved great success in combating a wide variety of disorders, it had not made much progress in curing other diseases, such as cancer, allergies, cardiovascular diseases, for example. At the same time, the existence of public concern about the side effects produced by prescribed drugs, doubt about the effectiveness of certain surgical operations, as well as the increasing costs of medical treatments, were constantly increasing.

A new wave of students was attracted by the philosophical precepts of the naturopathic medical profession, which encouraged appropriate use of science and showed interest in a modern university education and rising to the occasion. Bringing naturopathic medicine back into the medical mainstream required establishing accredited institutions, conducting credible research, and establishing itself as an integral part of the healthcare system.

In 1978 in the USA, the *John Bastyr College of Naturopathic Medicine* was established in Seattle, Washington, through Joseph E. Pizzorno, Jr. MD, Lestes E. Griffith, ND, William Mithell, MD and Sheila Quinn.

Its purpose was to teach scientifically based natural medicine, and thus, Bastyr became the first naturopathic college with accreditation. In 1993, in Arizona, Michael Cronnin, MD, and Conrad Kail, MD founded the *Southwest College of Naturopathic Medicine and Health Science*. With these first colleges accredited with active research and recognition of the appropriate application of science to natural medicine training and clinical practice, naturopathic medicine began to regain lost ground.

The disorders that increasingly prompt people, including physicians themselves, to explore unorthodox therapies are increasingly varied in both nature and severity:

- Degenerative cell diseases
- Chronic infections and allergies
- Anxiety, depression, migraines, insomnia
- Cancer and coronary heart disease
- Arthritis and other rheumatic disorders

All these diseases could be *relieved* by orthodox medicine in the mid-20th century, although it was not capable of *curing* them. In many cases, these reliefs produced side effects or reduced the patient's quality of life.

Unconventional therapies, or complementary, as they were also called, emphasize the fact that diseases are not the product of a single cause, but rather the combination of several factors:

- Hereditary predisposition
- Lifestyle and diet
- Mental and emotional state
- Spiritual state of the patient.

Many people who turn to complementary therapies do so after orthodox medicine has not been able to help them, and rheumatic patients, for example, were more willing to use them as their first option, especially osteopathy and chiropractic. In this way, the need to scientifically study some aspects of Alternative or Complementary Therapies began to arise. As science began to explore this need more and more, more and more conventional doctors began to employ some of the most promising techniques of Complementary Therapies. The clinical applications, as well as the results obtained through research in areas of Alternative Therapies, have earned a well-deserved place in orthodox medical journals.

It is no longer possible to maintain the traditional medical idea that it is unethical to recommend consultation with a complementary therapist, and the pressure exerted by both the public and medical organizations to include Complementary Therapy in the National Health Service, is growing. The World Health Organization (WHO) at its annual meeting in Geneva in 1990 declared:

"It is important and relevant to begin to consider the contribution that Non-Conventional Medicine is making in the field of Preventive Medicine.

It was urged that all public and private institutions dedicated to the field of health in each nation begin to promote, investigate and incorporate the different disciplines that make up Complementary Therapies into their health practice."

After the Geneva declaration of the WHO in 1990, there has been a significant rise in Complementary or Alternative Therapies on the 5 continents, as revealed by published statistics:

a.-Use of Non-Conventional Therapies by some countries (WHO 2005):

- United States: 45%
- Australia 48%
- France 49%
- Canada 70%
- India 70%
- Spain 30%
- Africa 80%

b.-Use of non-conventional therapies in the management of some health problems in the United States according to the National Institute of Health (NIH-2004):

- Patients with Chronic Sinusitis......81%
- Infected with HIV 50%
- Cancer Patients.........................63%
- Patients with Psoriasis................62%

- Patients with Lupus...................49%
- Children with Lymphoblastic Leukemia...40%
- Patients with organ transplant...............20%

c.-Consumption of unconventional therapy services and products in the United States in billions of dollars annually, published in the journal of the American Medical Association (JAMA-1998):

- Consultations with professionals $19.6
- Consumption of vitamins and minerals...........$4.7
- Consumption of dietary products.................$3.3
- Consumption of Herbal products................$5.1
- Annual total....................................$34.4

d.-Important university research centers were created to validate the scientific nature of non-conventional therapies in the most prestigious Medical Schools in the United States with an annual budget of $200 million:

- AIDS research center. Bastyr Univ. Washington. nineteen ninety-five
- Women's health research center. Columbia Univ. New York. 1993
- Research center for various medical conditions. Harvard 1993
- Neurological diseases research center. Kessler Univ. 1994
- Chiropractic research center. Palmer Univ. Davenport-Iowa. nineteen ninety-five
- Research center on the effect of age. Stanford 1994
- Research center in pediatric conditions. Arizona Univ. Tucson. nineteen ninety-six
- Asthma and immunology research center. Calf. Davis Univ. nineteen ninety-five
- Pain research center. Maryland Univ. Baltimore. 1997
- Research center for cardiovascular diseases. Michigan Univ.1996
- Addiction research center. Minnesota Univ. Minneapolis. nineteen ninety-five
- Cancer research center. Texas Univ. Houston. 1993

Although naturopathic doctors of the 19th century were astute clinical observers, they lacked the scientific tools to assess the validity of their concepts and showed little inclination to apply laboratory research, especially when science was frequently used to eliminate your profession.

During the last decade of the 20th century and the first decade of the 21st century, different research provided scientific documentation for most of the concepts of unconventional medicine, and the new generation of naturopathic medical scientists is using this research to continue the expansion of the profession.

Non-Conventional, alternative, or complementary Medicine, like the entire concept of Natural Medicine, may seem like an unscientific fad that will soon pass. For those who are informed, the new natural medicine leads the forefront of medicine of the future. The scientific tools that exist today allow us to evaluate and appreciate many aspects of natural medicine.

All of this illustrates the paradigm shift occurring within medicine, where what was once despised is being accepted as effective. In fact, in most cases, the natural alternative offers significant advantages over standard medical practices. In the future, the concepts, philosophies, and practices of unconventional medicines will become increasingly accepted. The practice of non-conventional medicines is rapidly growing, its therapeutic and diagnostic abilities are becoming increasingly sophisticated, and public interest is increasing. The crucial key to the future of this form of medicine is for it to become an integral part of the public healthcare system of most countries.

Non-Conventional Medicine of the 21st century is based on all the ancient principles forged by the great vitalist doctors of the past and that make up the solid paradigms that define it, which are:

a.-There is an internal force or power of *self-healing* that tends to keep the body in a state of health permanently and its ability to achieve this lies in the degree of physiological balance existing at each moment.

b.-The state of health of a person depends on the level of balance existing between physical, psychological, emotional, and social factors, therefore, any imbalance can cause loss of health. The human being achieves his balance to the extent that he respects the balance of natural laws.

c.-The naturopathic doctor must focus on looking for the *root* of the imbalances that his patient suffers, and once located, he must strive to implement the necessary changes in the lifestyle to correct these imbalances and promote with this is the restoration of health.

d.-Naturopathic medicine does not consider the human being divided or fractionated into zones, organs, or systems (reductionist approach), but conceives it as an integrated entity that works as a whole (holistic approach).

e.-In naturopathic medicine, health is the normal state of the human being, physical, psychological, and spiritual.

f.-Natural remedies must not cause harm to man, animals, and nature. They should be easy to understand and apply in most cases. Its effect must be pleasant and without creating any harm.

g.-Naturopathic medicine does not have specialties, it is based on a series of natural therapies to form a complete treatment.

h.-Naturopathic medicine preserves health with the means that nature offers, sun, water, air, earth, plants, food, exercise, and rest.

i.-The naturopathic doctor must first be a specialist in how to preserve health, and if it is lost, he must help cure it, using natural remedies. If healing is not possible, he must help alleviate the suffering; if nothing is possible, he must console.

j.- He must get the patient a positive attitude towards the disease, he must calm his patients, give them encouragement and fortitude so that they fight against his illness until he defeats it. Once the patient is healed, try to maintain healthy lifestyle habits.

k.-He must be aware that he is not the one who cures the sick, with his advice he helps an organism that fights the disease on its own and comes out of it.

In the first decade of the 21st century, a new trend in medicine has emerged called *Integrative Medicine*, defined as that practiced by a doctor, knowledgeable in conventional and non-conventional medicine (acupuncture, phytotherapy, naturopathy, nutritherapy, etc.), who promotes active participation of the person who comes to the consultation, in the process of searching for their physical, psychological and social well-being, accompanying them and guiding them in its development. It represents the last frontier in health services, which uses the available elements and therapies, based on scientific evidence, regardless of their source, to reverse the basic cause that generates the disease, increasing the state of well-being and health.

Integrative Medicine adds all forms of medicine and therapies, with a scientific basis, to achieve the best results for the patient. Includes:
- Conventional Medicine
- Mind – Body Medicine
- Emotion management
- Lifestyle, physical exercise, and nutrition
- Acupuncture, herbal medicine, massage
- Dentistry, biological and biophysical therapies
- Homeopathy and Homotoxicology.

By combining conventional medicine with preventive and non-conventional medicine, integrative medicine proposes a new way of practicing the art of health, promoting the conception of a *new patient,* open to change, responsible for their health and proactive in the process of preserving it; and a *new therapist,* empathetic, participatory, and willing to work as a team with the patient and other health professionals. The fundamentals or bases of integrative medicine include:

- An ancient paradigm of healing present in multiple cultures
- It is based on the concept of the human body's own healing process.
- Oriented more towards the reversal of the cause than towards the relief of the symptoms.
- Use the therapeutic resources that nature provides.
- Vis Medicatrix Natura: the healing power of nature.
- Primum Non Nocere: first do no harm.
- Tolle Causam: find the root cause.
- Treat the person in a comprehensive and complete manner.
- Preventive rather than curative medicine.
- Promotion of well-being and healthy lifestyles.
- Promotes education for health and well-being.
- The therapist is an educator and facilitator of the healing process
- Health is a positive state, not the absence of disease.
- Everyone is unique and constantly changing.
- Emphasizes individual responsibility in maintaining health.
- Health lies in the mind/body/spirit interaction.
- Individualizes diagnosis and treatment.
- Emphasizes the use of natural substances and restricts the use of synthetic ones.

As the 21st century progresses, more and more conventional doctors are interested in studying and practicing Integrative Medicine, motivated by different reasons:

- Discomfort and dissatisfaction with biomedicine and the pharmaceutical industry.
- Concern about the dangers inherent in conventional medical practice.
- Marketing with the needs of the community and patients.

- The acceptance that there are other effective and possible healing processes.
- Personal questioning as a professional of sometimes ineffective medicine.
- Transcend the limits of drugs and surgery as the only therapeutic tool.

Chapter 1

Pablo's Heart is not working well.

Pablo is a 45-year-old man, who lived alone in a rented apartment, had a very poor quality of life, had little strength to get around in his wheelchair, had permanent respiratory distress, and had swollen legs. He was taking several heart medications and was being observed and monitored with checkups every 6 months to see if he qualified to be placed on a Heart Transplant waiting list.

Pablo suffered from a genetic and hereditary disease called *Becker Muscular Dystrophy* that began to weaken his legs from the age of 20 until he was confined to a wheelchair at the age of 40. At the age of 30, the disease affected his heart, causing abnormal growth (*cardiomegaly*) with progressive loss of its strength (*heart failure*).

In March 2015 he had suffered a worsening of his heart and his lungs filled with fluid, a very delicate clinical condition called *Acute Lung Edema*, which required hospitalization for a week in intensive care and later hospitalization for 35 days. Due to a dangerous arrhythmia that he had; it was necessary to have a device called an *Automatic Implantable Defibrillator* (ICD) placed in his chest.

After leaving the hospital they gave him a medical report with the definitive diagnoses of his medical condition, which were as follows:

.-Grade IV dilated cardiomyopathy due to Becker Muscular Dystrophy

.-Congestive Heart Failure (CHF) class III

.-Severe Cardiac Arrhythmia controlled with ICD

.-Eventual candidate for heart transplant

The medical indication they gave him was to take medication based on diuretics (Furosemide and Aldactone) to prevent fluid retention and a vasodilator (Losartan) to keep blood pressure low and facilitate the work of the heart. They also told him that he had to go for a cardiological medical check-up every 6 months to perform tests and monitor his progress.

In September 2015, Pablo made his first visit to my office and brought with him the results of the last ultrasound that had been performed on his heart in June 2015, the results of which were as follows:

Echocardiogram June 2015:

- Left atrium: 40mm (maximum 35mm)
- Left ventricle: Diastole 68mm (maximum 46mm)
- Left ventricle: Systole 60mm (maximum 40mm)
- Ejection Fraction: 24% (normal 60% to 70%)
- Mitral valve: dilated and insufficient grade III
- Diagnosis: Severe dilated cardiomyopathy, CHF grade IV Mitral regurgitation grade III

On his first visit to my office, I asked Pablo what he thought about his illness and what his doubts were, and he told me that he had three main concerns, which were:

1-Am I condemned to live with respiratory distress, tachycardia, and swollen feet until I die?

2-My only hope for survival is a Heart Transplant??

3-Is there any other *alternative* that is less invasive and more hopeful

Pablo lived with fear and uncertainty about his future because his doctors had told him that he had a heart like that of a 90-year-old man and that his prognosis was *reserved*. Despite everything, he had the hope that there could be a solution for his heart, different from the one proposed by the doctors who treated him, and that belief was based on a book he was reading, (*How I Managed to Raise My Heart Ejection Fraction from 20% to 60%, by Alejandro Cienfuegos*) where the author told his own story, very similar to his, with a very enlarged heart and on the waiting list for a transplant, however, following medical treatments he did not based on nutrients and special supplements, he had managed to save himself from that fate, and miraculously recovered his heart to be able to lead a quality life.

I also asked Pablo what his expectations were and what he hoped to achieve by undergoing integrative medical treatment, that respected his normal medication and that gave him nutritional support and supplements for his heart. He told me that he had a series of questions that were constantly running through his mind, especially after having read the book. Those questions were:

- Is it possible to heal the heart?
- Is it possible to reduce the size of the heart?
- Is it possible to increase the strength of the heart?
- Are there natural treatments that can do it?
- Can a heart transplant be avoided?
- If this person achieved it; Could I do it too?

What does *Conventional Medicine* think?

Diseases of the heart muscle are included in the term cardiomyopathy. Among them, the most common is dilated cardiomyopathy, which is characterized by dilation and dysfunction of the left half of the heart, the right, or both. The prevalence of dilated cardiomyopathy in adults is 1 per 500 individuals and the causes include genetic or hereditary (20 to 48%), infections (viruses and parasites) and toxic (alcohol and cocaine).

The cause of Pablo's heart disorder is genetic, due to a disease called *Becker Muscular Dystrophy*, an inherited muscle disease caused by changes in the gene that controls the synthesis of *dystrophin*, a protein essential for normal muscle function. Patients with this disease present muscle atrophy and weakness.

In the heart, a lack of *dystrophin* causes muscle damage and scar tissue formation, which subsequently leads to heart failure. Over time, the chambers of the heart become larger, known as dilated cardiomyopathy. This serious complication can be fatal.

Despite the beneficial effect demonstrated in the latest clinical trials (CONSENSUS, RALES, SOLVD, CIBIS, MERIT-HF) the prognosis of chronic heart failure (CHF) in the general community has not yet improved substantially.

Dilated cardiomyopathy in its form of severe chronic heart failure can achieve high mortality, up to 50% 2 years after diagnosis. There is currently no cure for dilated cardiomyopathy, but treatment with medications helps control symptoms and reduces the risk of the disease getting worse or new symptoms developing.

Some people may need to have a pacemaker or ICD (implantable automatic defibrillator) implanted. In some cases, the option of a heart transplant may be considered. Heart transplantation probably offers, today, the best survival for subjects with severe CHF due to dilated cardiomyopathy. Unfortunately, the shortage of donors has not allowed it to increase above about 5,000 procedures per year, of which about 2,400 are performed in the United States. In the future, gene therapy and the use of stem cells may play an important role, as indicated by the lines of research currently open in this regard.

What does *Non-Conventional Medicine* think?

Research by Doctor Dean Ornish (1991) demonstrated that heart disease can be reversed with a diet that includes predominantly plant foods such as whole grains, fruits, vegetables, legumes, soy products, with the option of fat-free dairy and whites of egg.

Drawing on decades of research, Dr. Caldwell Esselstyn teaches us how to prevent and reverse heart disease, even in patients affected for years. His idea about the curative powers of proper nutrition in cases of heart disease has been proven true. Dr. Esselstyn has led pioneering research (2010) and has shown that the progression of heart disease, even severe, can be reversed by introducing comprehensive changes in diet and lifestyle.

Dr. Mathias Rath, 1995: Our research in cardiovascular diseases focuses on the beneficial health effects of essential vitamins and nutrients on various aspects of cardiovascular disease, its onset and gradual progression.

Most of the vital cellular nutrients essential for life cannot be produced by our body or only in insufficient quantities. To supply our body with vitamins and other cellular micronutrients, a balanced and varied diet is necessary. Nutritional supplementation with vitamins and other cellular micronutrients contributes to strengthening cellular metabolism.

Dr. Rath's Vital Cellular Nutrient Program offers cellular nutrient synergies for daily delivery, in a select variety of vitamins, minerals, trace minerals and other nutritional elements that are combined to support certain metabolic processes and restore heart health.

What was the treatment followed by Pablo?

Since September 2015 and for the following four years, Pablo followed a Heart-Healthy Eating scheme based on the principles established by Dr. Dean Ornish's program, which consisted of:

1.-Foods to avoid:

a.-Trans Fats

• Increase LDL oxidation, inflammation, endothelial dysfunction and atherogenesis

• Especially fried foods, fast foods, and hydrogenated fats

b.-Processed Meats or Sausages

• They increase the risk of heart attack by 40%

c.-Milk and Dairy Products

• They provide sodium, animal protein and saturated fat

• Contribute to the development of atherosclerosis

d.-Refined salt and sugar

• Sugar inflames the arteries and promotes their hardening

• Excess sodium chloride increases blood pressure

e.-Stimulant Drinks

• Coffee, mate, carbonated soft drinks.

• They increase the risk of arrhythmias and heart attack

f.-Alcoholic beverages:

• Alcohol damages the myocardium and generates cardiac arrhythmias

• Alcoholic Cardiomyopathy is common among habitual drinkers

2.-Recommended Foods

a.-Various Fruits

• Rich in vitamins, minerals, and phytochemicals

• Its antioxidant potential reduces the risk of heart attack

b.-Vegetables

• Its richness in vitamins and minerals helps prevent atherosclerosis

• Its contribution of potassium and magnesium exerts a regulating effect on blood pressure.

c.-Legumes

• They provide potassium, fiber, and B complex

• They help regulate blood pressure and avoid hypertension

d.-Whole Cereals

• They provide fiber, B complex and selenium

• Its effect is cardio nutritive and cardioprotective

e.-Nuts

• They provide vitamin E and antioxidants

• They provide unsaturated fatty acids

f.-Extra virgin Vegetable Oils

- They provide omega 3-6-9 fatty acids
- Reduce fibrinogen levels
- Prevent coronary heart disease

In addition to a heart-healthy eating plan, Pablo also followed a heart-healthy supplementation plan following the principles proposed by Dr. Mathias Rath. The following supplements were prescribed:

*-Magnesium (Mg) and Potassium (K)

.-Mg and K deficiency generates a proinflammatory, prothrombotic and proatherogenic environment that leads to endothelial dysfunction

.-Mg increases the energy of the heart, dilates the coronary arteries, reduces peripheral vascular resistance, inhibits platelet aggregation and coagulation.

.-Mg reduces the size of a heart attack, improves heart rate and reduces the incidence of cardiac arrhythmias.

.-Mg and K supplements are effective against angina, cardiac arrhythmias, CHF and high blood pressure.

*-Selenium

.-Low levels of selenium are associated with a greater risk of atherosclerosis

.-Exercises anti-atherogenic activity due to its antioxidant effect

.-Acts as a cofactor of the enzyme glutathione peroxidase which reduces the formation of hydrogen peroxide and lipid peroxidation.

*-Niacin (B3)

.-Decreases LDL by 16-23%, LP(a) by 35%, increases HDL by 20-33%

.-Reduces triglycerides, CRP and fibrinogen

.-It is the only natural lipid-lowering agent that has demonstrated a reduction in mortality

.-Its effects are long-lasting and gives better overall results than statins

*-Pyridoxine (B6), Cobalamin (B12), Folic Acid (B9)

.-The deficiency of B6, B9, B12 produces an increase in homocysteine in the blood

.-Homocysteine has atherogenic, prothrombotic and procoagulant properties

.-B6; 100mg/day. B12; 5000 mcg/day. Folate: 1mg/day prevents and normalizes homocysteine levels in the blood.

*-Vitamin C

.-Acts together with antioxidant enzymes: SOD, Catalase, Glutathione peroxidase

.-Strengthens arterial collagen, reduces CT, LP(a), BP, markers of inflammation and platelet aggregation, increases HDL and enhances fibrinolysis.

.-Prevents the oxidation of LDL, reduces the risk of MI and stroke

.-Decreases the standardized mortality ratio up to 48%, which is equivalent to an increase in longevity of 5-7 years in men and 1-3 years in women.

*-L-Taurine

.-Regulates the cellular excitability of cardiac tissue

.-Economizes the loss of potassium in the cardiac muscle

.-Regulates the osmotic control of calcium and potassium in the heart

.-Helps control blood cholesterol levels by improving its elimination

.-Antioxidant, anti-atherogenic, lipid-lowering, hypotensive.

*-L-Carnitine

.-Improves lipid metabolism in the heart

.-Reduces total cholesterol and triglyceride levels

.-Prevents the development of coronary heart disease and angina pectoris

.-Prevents the appearance of cardiac arrhythmias

How did Pablo evolve with this treatment?

The medical check-ups were rigorous every 3 months, and we were both able to see a progressive improvement in all the clinical symptoms and the most surprising thing is that his heart was reducing in size significantly. Mitral valve dysfunction has also improved substantially. And the Ejection Fraction or Heart Force has risen to 49% in 4 years of treatment.

The result of the last ultrasound of the heart that Pablo brought us showed the following values:

Echocardiogram April 2019

- Left atrium: 35 mm
- Left Ventricle: Diastole 57 mm
- Left ventricle: Systole 51 mm
- Ejection Fraction: 49%
- Mitral: good opening and minimal insufficiency
- Diagnosis: Mild dilated cardiomyopathy, CHF grade I and Mitral Insufficiency grade I.

Conclusions

1.-This story illustrates with well-documented details that the response capacity of the human organism is simply *surprising* when it is provided with the necessary and adequate resources.

2.-The *truths* of *Conventional Medicine* are limited by the procedures and techniques of this Medicine, but at no time do they reflect 100% of reality.

3.-The combination of a *Heart-Healthy Diet and Supplementation* rigorously followed by the patient and opportunely controlled and monitored by the doctor, can achieve surprising results like the one our patient obtained.

4.-It was possible to *Revert* a condition of Severe Left Heart Failure to a new condition of Mild Left Heart Failure.

5.-The results obtained were evidenced, both in the clinical evolution of the patient, who managed to significantly improve his level and quality of life in 4 years of treatment, and in the Chest X-rays and Echocardiogram that recorded the reduction in the diameters of the cavities of the heart and the increase in the Ejection Fraction, which went from 24% in May 2015 to 49% in April 2019

6.-There is no conventional medical publication that demonstrates similar results, to those obtained in this case, following standard pharmacological treatments for this type of pathology.

7.-Based on this experience, it is highly recommended that all patients suffering from cardiovascular pathology be incorporated into a complementary regimen of *Cardio healthy* Food and Supplementation following the guidelines established by Doctors Dean Ornish and Mathias Rath, since their works are widely supported scientifically.

Discussion

When a person who suffers from *Muscular Dystrophy* (Duchenne or Becker), their heart is damaged, becoming progressively large (*cardiomegaly*) and weak (*heart failure*), with a progressive loss of its strength, go to the Cardiology Service, public or private, in search of a solution to this problem. The patient undergoes special tests (*Ultrasound, Holter for arrhythmias, MRI of the heart*) to determine the magnitude of the damage to the heart, establish the degree of cardiomegaly and insufficiency on a scale from I to IV, and then determine the most appropriate treatment. to achieve the ideal objectives, which in these cases are:

a.-Control symptoms such as cough, respiratory distress, fluid retention in the lungs and lower extremities, palpitations, tachycardia, or any other type of arrhythmia.

b.-Avoid complications such as heart collapse that leads to *Acute pulmonary edema* or sudden loss of consciousness due to *Syncope*, two situations that usually threaten the patient's life.

c.-Determine if the patient meets criteria for the placement of a pacemaker (PM) or an implantable automatic defibrillator (ICD), to avoid sudden death due to the presence of malignant arrhythmias.

d.-Try to prolong life in a pathology (*dilated cardiomyopathy*) that even today has a very poor prognosis, with a mortality of 50% in the first 2 years after the diagnosis.

e.-In the best of cases, if it is not possible to control the symptoms and complications, due to the progression of the disease, determine if the patient qualifies for an eventual *Heart Transplant* as a final solution in the search to preserve life.

For *Conventional Medicine*, dilated cardiomyopathy is an *incurable* disease that progresses towards frequent complications and high short-term mortality, and only heart transplantation offers hope. These are *iron truths* for *Conventional Medicine* and cardiologists who treat these types of patients never consider the possibility that there are other solutions different from those established by world-renowned cardiological institutions such as the *American Heart Association* (AHA), the *American Heart College* (ACC) and the *European Heart Institute* (IEC).

Patients who suffer from this medical condition complain that their treating doctors do not dedicate time to them in follow-up consultations (10 to 20 minutes), they limit themselves to performing the required tests (ultrasound, Holter, etc.), they do not offer them any explanation nor do they tell them anything about the state of the disease, its evolution and prognosis, they get upset if they are asked any questions and patients in general feel that for their doctors they are *lost cases* in which it is not worth wasting time and effort, limiting themselves to the established minimum, the required medications, special tests and then giving them an appointment for six months or a year.

Hippocrates, the father of Western medicine, points out in his Hippocratic Oath that: *"the fundamental and primary task of the doctor is to preserve life whenever possible."* The manual of the International Rights of patients and all the official texts on the Code of Ethics and Medical Deontology that are edited and defended by all Western Medical Colleges and Federations point out that:

"Every patient has the right to receive the best scientifically proven medical treatment to improve their symptoms and eventually cure their illness; and the doctor is obliged to stay as updated as possible to be able to ensure compliance with this mandate for his patient."

Doctors and researchers Dean Ornish and Mathias Rath are professionals who studied and graduated from recognized universities in their countries of origin, received the medical degree provided by the faculty of practicing medicine, are registered in the required Medical Colleges and meet all national and international standards to practice your profession. Both ventured into medical research in the field of cardiology.

Dr. Dean Ornish did so by relating healthy eating to recovery from coronary heart disease (1981), and Dr. Mathias Rath did so by relating nutritional supplementation to recovery from coronary heart disease, high blood pressure, and other cardiovascular diseases (1985). Both doctors presented the results of their research at world medical conferences organized by the American Heart Association, the American College of the Heart, the Preventive Medicine Association, and the Orthomolecular Medicine Association, and have also published articles in scientific medical journals of world order and have written books where they have presented their experiences, studies and results.

It is appropriate to ask then:

Why do most Western doctors in general, and cardiologists in particular, ignore the work of these two eminent and renowned doctors and researchers who have dedicated their lives, efforts, sacrifices and resources to work and scientifically demonstrate that it is possible to help patients affected by cardiovascular disease to recover and even heal, without the need to use drugs or surgery, and by only applying a heart-healthy diet and supplementation following the guidelines established by their research?

It is also appropriate to ask:

Why do doctors who do know the work of these researchers not apply their recommendations and treatments to benefit their patients, even though these investigations were carried out following all scientific standards and have been accepted by the world medical community of all countries?

It is no secret that the pharmaceutical chemical industry controls, through economic and financial agreements, most, if not all, world-renowned medical institutions, and associations, even reaching the offices of the World Health Organization, exercising a dangerously important influence in the direction and policy of all these institutions.

Considering this terrible but crude truth, it is not surprising then that most doctors and cardiologists in the world ignore or despise the truths demonstrated by other medical researchers who have based their work on *natural or non-pharmacological* topics.

Simply because this research do not are aligned with the economic interests of the powerful pharmaceutical chemical industry.

On the other hand, the majority of conventional doctors who work and fight in official clinics and hospitals are practically *hypnotized* by the chemical pharmaceutical industry, who, using an excessively materialist and Cartesian discourse and dialectic, cunningly disguised as scientific, has made to believe that they and only they are the bearers of the only truth, to which doctors must blindly adhere and defend, rejecting everything that does not come from their headquarters, and all of this supported by the World Health Organization.

Chapter 2

Ruth's Red Spots

Ruth is a 57-year-old schoolteacher who began suffering from a skin disorder in January 2017. Suddenly, red spots began to appear in different parts of her body. They were painful, stinging and burning, they had different sizes and shapes, some confluent and with different shades. The spots lasted three to five days and disappeared spontaneously.

The episodes occurred every two to three weeks and at first, they only appeared in her arms, then the episodes became more frequent and extensive, covering her legs, trunk and finally her face. The situation reached the point of having to rest at home on the days that she had the spots, because they were very annoying, and because they gave her a very unpleasant appearance and since she worked with children, she could not do it in those conditions.

From the first episode, Ruth went to her primary care doctor who interpreted it as an allergy and tried several treatments with anti-allergy medication, which were unsuccessful and did not solve the problem. In March 2017 Ruth was referred to Dermatology, she received a couple of treatments based on creams, body lotions and other anti-allergy medications, which were also not effective.

When the dermatologist saw the patient with the lesions, she concluded that it was *Erythema Multiforme* and told him that she should undergo a treatment based on *cortisone*, an intramuscular injection every 3 weeks.

Because Ruth was desperate, she accepted the cortisone-based treatment and the result of the first injection was fabulous, as the spots disappeared within 8 to 10 hours.

After having received 4 successive doses of cortisone, the effect of which lasted only about three weeks, after which the spots reappeared, Ruth noticed that she had gained 10 kg, that her blood pressure rose to values that required medication and she is now Her blood glucose was rising, putting her at risk of becoming diabetic, all caused by the cortisone. Because of this, Ruth asked her dermatologist how long the cortisone treatment would last, and her doctor answered:

"Well, you have to make a decision, either you continue with cortisone to stay free of Erythema Multiforme, despite the side effects, which in any case we can control with other medications, or you stop cortisone and return to your frequent attacks of Erythema Multiform".

Ruth visited me on 07/01/2017 and stated that she was in a medical trap, because if she continued applying the cortisone injection, to improve her Erythema Multiforme outbreak, she had to endure the annoying and dangerous side effects that this caused. medication. And if cortisone was not applied, I would have to endure outbreaks of Erythema Multiforme, which are also very unpleasant and limiting. Once she explained her dilemma and her anguish, she asked the following two questions:

*-Is there any solution for this crossroads?

*-Is there a solution for *Erythema Multiforme* outbreak other than cortisone injection?

What does Conventional Medicine think?

Erythema Multiforme is a rare, acute skin and mucosal reaction. It is a hypersensitivity reaction, characterized by target-shaped skin eruptions, made up of concentric areas of different color, and ulcerative lesions or lesions in the form of vesicles or blisters on the mucosa, such as the mouth or nose. They are acute, self-limiting injuries that resolve in 3-4 weeks, are very painful and significantly alter the patient's general condition.

Many suspected etiological factors have been reported to cause this skin disorder, the most common being the following list of such factors:

*-Bacterial infections: streptococcus, legionella, Neisseria, Mycobacteria (leprosy and tuberculosis), salmonella, etc.

*-Fungi: Coccidioides immitis

*-Parasites: toxoplasma and Trichomonas

*-Medicines: antibiotics (penicillin and sulfonamides), aspirin, anticonvulsants (phenobarbital and phenytoin)

*- Physical factors: radiotherapy, cold, sunlight.

*-Other diseases: vasculitis, Hodgkin lymphoma, leukemia, multiple myeloma, polycythemia.

Erythema Multiforme resolves spontaneously, most of the time, so treatment is usually unnecessary. Corticosteroids and topical anesthetics and oral antihistamines can improve symptoms and calm patients.

Recurrences are common, and empirical maintenance treatment with antiherpetic drugs such as acyclovir 400 mg orally every 12 hours, famciclovir 250 mg orally every 12 hours, or valacyclovir 1,000 mg orally every 24 hours may be indicated if symptoms recur. more than 5 times a year and an association with the herpes simplex virus is suspected or if recurrent erythema multiforme is always preceded by outbreaks of herpes infection.

What does non-conventional medicine think?

The skin often expresses what happens inside the body. Talking about a skin-gut connection may seem surprising at first glance. However, the integrative approach to medicine proposes going beyond the specific specialties that address the disease from a single organ to establish an interdisciplinary connection. Whether we have itching, pimples, dermatitis or psoriasis, many times the explanation for all these phenomena lies beyond the skin itself, and the intestine has a lot to say on this topic. Let's examine the issue a little.

The intestine was considered mechanical for many years. A simple tube through which food passed before being excreted. But during the 20th century, many lines of research appeared, and many amazing functions were discovered. All of this in constant review and updating. To round out the concept we can say that in the intestine there are four important actors:

- The cells that line the intestinal tube on the inside: the mucosa
- Intestinal bacteria: the flora or Microbiota
- The intestinal immune system
- The Enteric Nervous System

The **Mucosa** forms a countless series of folds called villi. It does this to increase the absorption surface in a smaller space. However, if we stretched all those villi, it would be equal to the surface of a tennis court! (300 square meters). And why is it so important that there is such a large surface area? For better absorption of the nutrients that come with food. In the small intestine this is of crucial importance, so much so that the thickness of the mucosa is restricted to a single layer of cells. Each intestinal cell is attached to the next by a kind of glue, so that the nutrients do not strain through the cracks but rather pass through the cell from top to bottom. And this is because each cell is a small factory that processes food to release it into circulation in the appropriate form. So, when the glue is damaged, unprocessed nutrients leak into the circulation, causing distant problems: joint pain, headaches, skin problems. This is what is called *leaky gut syndrome.*

The **Microbiota** is the name given to the bacteria that live in the intestine. We have 10 times more bacteria than cells, and in fact they can account for up to 2 kg of the total weight of an adult and constitute 50% of the feces. This microbiota is constantly studied and revised, with new functions continually being discovered within the human body. There are more than 500 different species of bacteria, of which 30 to 40 species predominate. When the proportion of intestinal bacteria is altered and unbalanced, dysbiosis appears, which causes many digestive discomforts such as bloating, gas, constipation, or diarrhea.

The *Intestinal Immune System*. Although it is not a well-known fact, the truth is that the intestine is responsible for 60 to 70% of our immune cells.

There are different specialized immune structures with the sole mission of protecting the body. It is logical since many substances penetrate through the digestive tract and the immune system must constantly monitor. When it is unbalanced, many diseases can appear allergies, repeated infections due to low defenses, autoimmune diseases, etc.

The *Enteric Nervous System*, known as the second brain, which has millions of neurons and neurotransmitters, substances that act as messengers capable of influencing mood and health. Among the neurotransmitters we find dopamine, serotonin, and histamine. Many depressive, anxiety and irritation states can be related to a deficiency or excess of these neurotransmitters. For example: when a person is constipated, they produce less serotonin and therefore may be prone to emotional disturbances. This is what is called the *brain-gut connection*.

And what is the relationship of some skin diseases with the intestine?

Mucosal alterations, such as the leaky gut syndrome, can be associated with conditions such as acne, rosacea, psoriasis, or atopic dermatitis. In fact, it is well documented that some psoriasis patients may be celiac or have gluten intolerance, which causes suffering and inflammation of the intestinal mucosa.

Alterations in the microbiota can cause dysbiosis due to proteolytic bacteria. These bacteria have the potential to manufacture biogenic amines, the most famous of which is histamine, which in high quantities can cause itching and rashes or aggravate conditions such as atopic dermatitis, psoriasis, and rosacea.

Alterations of the intestinal immune system can aggravate or induce allergic conditions, atopic dermatitis, and autoimmune diseases.

Alterations in the second brain explain many mood states that can accompany some skin diseases: depressive states, irritability, anxiety, etc.

That's why the integrative approach is so important and considering all the patient's symptoms, beyond the skin, because they often respond to the same imbalance that must be corrected. When this is the case, correcting intestinal disorders can improve some skin diseases and certain mood states that accompany them.

What was the treatment followed by Ruth?

In Ruth's medical history, some factors were detected that could be related to the appearance of the episodes of Erythema Multiforme that she had been suffering from for 6 months. These factors were:

a.-Chronic constipation associated with digestive dyspepsia and some food intolerances.

b.-Chronic stress with frequent anxiety episodes related to your workload

c.-Cigarette consumption, 1 box/day (20 cigarettes) for 15 years

d.-Consumption of 20 cups of coffee and 12 glasses of wine per month.

e.-Consumption of sweets, sauces, spicy foods, seafood, and pastries in excess.

f.-Chronic sedentary lifestyle and overweight of 20 kg.

g.-High cholesterol (268), low vitamin D3 (20), high Transaminase (GGT; 107) and low vitamin B12 (208).

A treatment scheme based on a lifestyle change, detoxification, nutritional education, and specific supplementation was proposed to Ruth to recover the nutritional deficiencies observed.

a.-Correct combination of foods, increase consumption of raw vegetables, whole grains, fresh seasonal fruits, and various seeds. Elimination of sauces, spicy foods, sweets, alcohol, coffee, and pastries.

b.-Treatment scheme to quit smoking, which was effective from the first week. She was also recommended a Yoga and Pilates program to regulate stress.

c.-You were given a simple exercise plan, walking 45 minutes a day in the evening.

d.-A liver detoxification plan based on vitamins, amino acids, and specific medicinal plants

e.-Correction using natural supplements of your cholesterol, vitamin D3 and vitamin B12 values.

How did Ruth evolve with this treatment?

After completing 3 months with the hygienic-dietary regimen, vitamin supplementation and medicinal plants, the results obtained were the following:

a.-Normalization of all laboratory parameters that were altered

b.-Reduction of 10 kg in weight

c.-Regulation of intestinal transit

d.-Disappearance of the episodes of "Erythema Multiforme" from the second week after starting the treatment.

Ruth remained free of Erythema Multiforme outbreaks from the second week after starting the integrative treatment and remained healthy for the next 28 months. Her last consultation was in November 2019, when she was discharged.

Conclusion

The skin is an organ that is part of the so-called *Tegumentary System* which also includes all the mucous membranes (digestive, respiratory, and genitourinary) and all the serous membranes (pleura, pericardium, and peritoneum).

All mucous membranes and the skin are interrelated through the large lymphoid system that they all have, forming the so-called MALT system (*mucosal associated lymphoid tissue*). Therefore, we cannot see the skin as an organ isolated from the rest of the body and whenever it is sick, with problems of dermatitis, eczema and other disorders, we must always look for the cause in the MALT system of mucosa, and treat any of them that is altered, since many times the lesions observed on the skin are nothing more than a distant manifestation of that diseased mucosa, which is almost always the digestive mucosa, as it has the largest surface area and the most exposed to the outside as it is in permanent contact with food and drinks.

In Ruth's case we work with this hypothesis, based on this anatomical and physiological fact, we treat her MALT mucosal system, specifically her digestive system, with a hygienic-dietary plan, detoxification and use of medicinal plants and natural supplements, achieving a highly satisfactory result that returned the patient to the functional normality of her skin and freed her from the need to use cortisone indefinitely.

It was also possible to prevent the progression of the side effects caused by this medication and which were already present in the patient at the time of coming to our consultation.

Discussion

The Specialization of conventional medicine proposes a professional exercise that *Fragments* the human being into many separate parts and specialist doctors confine themselves to treating only and exclusively the organ of the body that is the object of their specialty, to such an extent that it seems that they forget that this organ does not exist separately and independently from the rest of the organism, but on the contrary, each organ of the human body is closely related to all the other organs to form a large system that works as an integrated whole to maintain bodily homeostasis. and health status. Approaching medical practice under the approach of *super specialization* forgetting that we are an indivisible whole, connected on a molecular, biochemical, energetic, functional, and anatomical level, is an error in approach that will lead to obtaining unsatisfactory results.

If the human organism functions in an integrated way, similar to a symphony orchestra where each musician and each instrument contributes the magic of its sound to make it possible for the resulting melody to be the melody of health; In the same way we must give an integrated healing response to keep each organ functioning in harmony in its interaction with all the other organs, when the orchestra is out of tune or generating a melody of illness. Just as it is not the separate sound of the piano, violin or bass that generates the final melody of the orchestra, nor is it the separate functioning of a heart, kidney or liver that generates the state of homeostasis and health, but rather the harmonic sum of all organs functioning correctly.

If a dermatologist focuses on treating a skin disease as if that disease were the exclusive property of the skin, forgetting about the physiological and biochemical relationship of the skin with the rest of the body, he or she will never be able to get to the root of the disorder at hand reflecting on the skin, but not residing in it. In the case we have presented, the *Erythema Multiforme* that Ruth had been presenting for 6 months was not an exclusive and separate disease of the skin but was a distant manifestation of a functional disorder of the intestine and liver, which were overloaded with toxins and generating internal congestion that affected the skin.

For this reason, none of the treatments applied to the skin gave the expected results and it was only when the homeostatic functioning of the digestive and hepatobiliary system was restored, through a detoxification process and balanced diet, that complete improvement of the symptom was achieved.

It reflected the skin as *Erythema Multiforme*, and which was maintained over time in response to the healthy changes that the patient assumed responsibly.

When the patient had been receiving a monthly dose of intramuscular cortisone for 4 months, because it was the only medication that relieved her symptoms, without causing complete healing, the secondary symptoms of said medication began to appear, and the patient became concerned when she realized that her quality of life and health entered a spiral of deterioration, by increasing blood pressure, blood sugar, gaining weight, etc. and when she expressed this concern to her treating dermatologist, she, far from seeking a solution to the problem she was experiencing, posing her patient, and for whom she was largely responsible, she simply told the patient :

"Well, you have to make a decision, either you continue with cortisone to stay free of Erythema Multiforme, despite the side effects, which in any case we can control with other medications, or you stop cortisone and return to your frequent attacks of Erythema Multiforme".

Some questions arise that we can ask ourselves to understand the behavior that this doctor had with the patient:

* Why didn't she refer her to another doctor who could provide a different solution than the one she was offering the patient and who had placed her in a highly pressing dilemma since she was presenting delicate side effects?

* Maybe the doctor thought that if she referred the patient to another doctor, she was letting it be known that she was not able to solve the problem efficiently and that could call into question her prestige?

* Was the doctor afraid or reluctant to accept that she was not offering a satisfactory solution to this patient and on the contrary was causing other problems that were already distressing to the patient?

*Why does a specialist doctor choose to subject his patient to greater suffering, maintaining a medication that not only does not solve the problem of his illness definitively, but also causes other worse problems?

*Where were those promises of *commitment, compassion, understanding* and *maximum scientific effectiveness* that the doctor should offer to his patient, following the mandate of the deontological and ethical code that every doctor should profess?

When a specialist doctor forgets the principle of integration under which the human body functions and practices his profession in a fragmented way, focusing on treating isolated organs, and also subjects his patient to the tyranny of the misuse of pharmacology, thinking only of safeguard their prestige and their deified position before the patient and society; We must reflect on the paths that medicine is taking today and on the deep crisis that it is suffering in its core that leads it to violate its fundamental Hippocratic principles, such as the principle of *First do no harm* and the principle of *safeguard health and life at all costs.*

It is not acceptable, under any circumstances, for doctors, regardless of their philosophy, orthodox, conventional, complementary, non-conventional, etc., to continue practicing medicine that is distant and alien to the basic principles of ancient *Hippocratic philosophy* and based on evidence. scientific, since by continuing like this, far from fulfilling its beneficent role for a hurt and suffering humanity, it will be siding with the social agents that cause harm to human beings.

Chapter 3

Teresa suffers at mealtime.

Teresa is a 46-year-old woman with a long history of digestive disorders since she was 10 years old, having suffered from Intestinal Parasitosis, Hiatal Hernia, Helicobacter Pillory and Intestinal Candidiasis. In the last 6 years she has had very poor digestive health, because she always suffers from gas, abdominal bloating, colic, digestive heaviness, nausea, acid reflux and she has also noticed that many foods do not agree with her, to the point of tormenting herself every time who sits at the table at mealtime because she doesn't know what food she could eat that wouldn't cause the annoying symptoms she always has. Her family and friends see her as the strange one in the family because she is always complaining about food and digestive discomfort, to the point of affecting her social life, because no one wants to share celebrations and meetings around the table with someone. who can't eat almost anything.

As if that were not enough, Teresa not only suffers from her poor digestive health, but also from other health problems, which she firmly believes are related to her poor digestion, because in the past, when her digestion was good, she did not have those issues. First there were migraines, which started at 15 years of age, then respiratory allergies and asthma, which appeared at 25 years of age, and more recently, for the last 3 years, she has been suffering from recurrent urinary infections 5 episodes per year in the last 3 years.

Teresa has made a true pilgrimage through countless medical offices, and thus, in her search for a solution for her various health problems, she has visited gastroenterologists, neurologists, allergists, pulmonologists and urologists, and despite complying with all kinds of medication, which these doctors have indicated to her on multiple occasions, her symptoms, far from improving, are getting worse and worse, and for that reason, Teresa feels disappointed, frustrated and with little hope of finding a solution to her health problems.

Teresa visited me in May 2019 with the results of a gastroscopy and colonoscopy that had been performed 6 months ago, with no evidence of any disease that would explain the digestive symptoms that she constantly reported. The digestive doctor told her that she suffered from *Irritable Colon* and that she should be evaluated by a psychiatrist to resolve her problem. Recommendation that she did not follow and in her place, she considered looking for a different solution to see if she had better luck.

What does Conventional Medicine think?

Irritable colon, whose more accurate name is *Irritable Bowel Syndrome* (IBS), is a chronic and relapsing condition, characterized by the existence of abdominal pain and/or changes in intestinal rhythm (diarrhea or constipation). It may or may not be accompanied by a sensation of abdominal distension, without demonstrating an alteration in intestinal morphology or metabolism, or infectious causes that justify it. The precise cause of IBS is unknown, although a set of factors have been observed that seem to influence its origin, the most common being the following:

*-Intestinal infection: IBS can be triggered after having suffered an episode of gastroenteritis and is usually associated with bacterial overgrowth in the small intestine (SIBO).

*-Imbalance of the Microbiota: a modification of the bacteria that normally live in the colon (dysbiosis) can generate a series of disorders that end in IBS.

*-Intestinal inflammation: it has been observed that people who suffer from IBS have a strong reactivity of the intestinal immune system with elevation of certain inflammation markers present in the feces, such as calprotectin and lactoferrin.

*-Nervous disorders: people with IBS usually have certain nervous disorders that affect their digestive health and for this reason, intestinal symptoms are more common in times of stress.

The symptoms of irritable bowel syndrome (IBS) are usually triggered by certain factors that are common among people who suffer from it, such as:

*-Food: Many people have worse IBS symptoms when they eat or drink certain foods or drinks, such as wheat, dairy products, citrus fruits, beans, cabbage, milk, and carbonated drinks.

*-Hormones: it has been observed that most women who suffer from IBS tend to have more symptoms on the days of menstruation.

*-Mood disorders: It is very common for people who suffer from IBS to suffer from anxiety and depression.

There is no test to definitively diagnose IBS. Your doctor will likely begin with a complete medical history, physical examination, and tests to rule out other conditions. If you have diarrhea, you will likely be tested for gluten intolerance (celiac disease).

Once other conditions have been ruled out, your doctor will likely use the so-called Rome Criteria which include:

- Pain and discomfort lasting at least one day a week in the last three months
- Abdominal pain and discomfort usually improve with defecation
- The frequency of defecations is altered, it may alternate between diarrhea and constipation
- The consistency of bowel movements has changed and may contain mucus

Your doctor may order several tests to rule out other possible disorders that are related to your symptoms. Those tests may be some or all the following:

*-Stool analysis: to detect bacteria or parasites that may cause an intestinal infection

*-Gastroscopy: to investigate celiac disease or bacterial overgrowth

*-Colonoscopy: to examine the entire length of the colon for inflammation, tumors, or diverticula.

Treatment of irritable bowel syndrome focuses on relieving symptoms so that the person can live as normally as possible. Mild signs and symptoms can often be relieved by managing stress and making changes to your diet and lifestyle. The doctor usually advises:

- Avoid foods that trigger your symptoms
- Eat foods rich in fiber
- Drink much liquid
- Exercise regularly
- Get enough sleep

Although there are no specific medications to treat irritable bowel syndrome, it is common for your doctor to recommend a combination of drugs to relieve symptoms, such as:

*-Laxatives: to fight constipation

*-Anti diarrheal: to control the seasons of liquid evacuations

*-Anti spasmodic: to calm colic, cramps or intestinal cramps

*-Anti depressants: for depressed people with irritable bowel symptoms

*-Antibiotics: in case the existence of SIBO is proven

What does non-conventional medicine think?

Food intolerance is the difficulty that the body has in digesting certain foods. This causes certain reactions that arise shortly after ingesting them. The most common symptoms include: excess gas, abdominal pain or bloating, nausea, and other extra-digestive symptoms such as allergies. , migraine or joint and muscle pain. Foods most likely to cause these types of symptoms include milk, eggs, chocolate, bread, shrimp, and tomatoes, but many others can cause these types of signs, varying greatly from person to person.

Food intolerance affects each person differently and foods that benefit one person can be harmful to another. Therefore, it is necessary to analyze each case through a personalized clinical study.

To verify that it is a food intolerance, a series of specific tests must be carried out to identify which foods and nutrients cause the intolerance. The best-known tests are:

.-IgG Food Intolerance Test (ALCAT): The test is based on a simple blood draw, which is used to determine how the patient's antibodies react to certain protein substances present in food. Subsequently, an interpretation of the results carried out by medical professionals helps you know which the most appropriate diet is to keep your digestive health in perfect condition.

.-Exhaled air or breath test: It is recommended as a diagnostic guidance test in the event of suspected carbohydrate malabsorption and/or bacterial overgrowth, mainly. The breath test detects unabsorbed carbohydrates, so it could be considered an indicator of the digestive capacity of the small intestine. Currently this test is applied to detect malabsorption and intolerance to lactose, fructose, glucose, and lactulose. It has also been applied to people who are sensitive to sorbitol, a sugar derived from alcohol used in chewing gum, in diet products and as a sweetener in sugar-free pastries.

Dysbiosis or intestinal dysbacteriosis is a term that denotes a microbial imbalance or maladaptation within the body of an impaired microbiota. For example, a part of the human microbiota, such as the skin, intestinal or vaginal microbiota, can become disordered, with normally dominant species decreased and normally non-dominant species increased. Dysbiosis is most reported as a condition in the gastrointestinal tract, particularly during small intestine bacterial overgrowth (SIBO) or small intestine fungal overgrowth (SIFO).

The deterioration or imbalance of the intestinal microbiota is usually related to a series of factors specific to the individual or their relationship with the environment. In this sense, the following elements have been described:

*-Modern diet: excess of fast sugars, excess of proteins and fats

*-Insufficient chewing of food

*-Lack of digestive enzymes

*-Gastrointestinal infections: gastroenteritis and parasitosis

*-Antibiotics, chemotherapy, and radiotherapy

*-Chronic stress

To diagnose intestinal dysbiosis, it is necessary to perform a test to study the digestive microbiota through specialized analysis of a stool sample. Currently there are two modalities of this type of test, the one based on C-Reactive Protein, which is not very precise, and the one based on the Metagenomic study, which is much more accurate and safer. Unfortunately, this type of test is not performed by hospital or private laboratories, nor is it covered by most medical insurance, its cost is usually high ($400) and most conventional doctors are unaware of it or do not give it any importance; For all these reasons, intestinal dysbiosis usually goes unnoticed in most cases.

Intestinal dysbiosis must be treated to avoid the possible complications that it may cause in the future, not only in the digestive tract, but in the rest of the body. Those complications are:

*-Hormonal imbalance: we know that certain bacteria promote a hormonal imbalance.

*-Autoimmune diseases show clear links to the excessive growth of some bacteria.

*-Joint aches and pains can be caused by leaky gut, which is generally a consequence of some type of imbalance in the gastrointestinal microbiota.

*-Neurological and psychiatric diseases can be traced back to problems with our microbes.

*-Resistance to weight loss is often a consequence of bacterial overgrowth.

What was the treatment and evolution that Teresa followed?

Teresa underwent the food intolerance test (ALCAT) and the exhaled breath test, which was positive for malabsorption and intolerance to Lactose and Sorbitol, for this reason she was recommended to eat a diet free of all foods that They contain lactose and sorbitol. As a result, in a few weeks most of the digestive symptoms that she had been experiencing for years disappeared.

Once the diagnosis of food intolerance was established and verified, identifying the foods and sugars responsible for said intolerance, the next step was to carry out an *Advanced Study of Intestinal Health* to evaluate the primary cause that was causing said problem.

That is, identify the specific element of her intestinal ecosystem that was affected and that was responsible for the food intolerances detected. The advanced gut health study included:

a.-Microbiota test; to investigate whether there was intestinal dysbiosis

b.-Test of Fecal Zonulin; to investigate if there was Leaky Gut

c.-Test of Fecal Calprotectin; to investigate if there was intestinal inflammation

d.-Test of Pancreatic Elastase to investigate if there was a deficiency of digestive enzymes

e.-IgA anti-gliadin and anti-endomysium test to evaluate Celiac disease

The results of all these tests were the following:

*Mild deficiency of the Immune Microbiota with a decrease in *Enterococcus* strains

*Mild deficiency of the Nutritive Microbiota with a decrease in *Faecalibacterium* strains

*Moderate deficiency of the Protective Microbiota with a decrease in *Lactobacilli* strains

*Significant increase in *Candida Albicans* type yeasts

With this result, the final diagnosis of Dysbiosis and Intestinal Candidiasis was reached, and it was considered that this is the logical consequence of a long history of taking medications and the reason for the food intolerances that Teresa had suffered for six years.

After nine months of treatment based on a diet free of fermentative sugars, especially lactose and sorbitol, to reduce the symptoms of food intolerance, in addition to Probiotics, Prebiotics, Butyric Acid to restore and balance the microbiota intestinal, eliminating the dysbiosis found, and Caprylic Acid and Palo de Arco to treat intestinal candidiasis, Teresa managed to achieve an improvement in all her digestive and extra-digestive symptoms, thereby improving her quality of life significantly.

Conclusion

Based on the data provided by this patient in her clinical history, it was easy to consider that she most likely had an alteration in her intestinal ecosystem because of so many digestive disorders suffered throughout her life.

Such as gastroesophageal reflux, which required medication with omeprazole, intestinal parasitosis, which required medication with antiparasitic drugs, helicobacter pylori, which required treatment with antibiotics; In addition, all the drugs indicated for her migraine, rhinitis, bronchial asthma, and urinary infections problems.

Given the intake of so many drugs throughout her life, it was to be assumed that she would most likely have an alteration of the digestive microbiota, called *Intestinal Dysbiosis*, which in turn led to an alteration of the digestive processes, causing malabsorption of nutrients and food intolerances, which in fact she had accused for years. As has been reported in the medical literature, food intolerances are manifested by digestive symptoms, like all those the patient had, but they can also present with extra-digestive or systemic symptoms, many of which were also present in this case, such as migraine, respiratory allergies, and urinary infections.

It is a clear case of *Mucous Disease* due to an affectation of the mucous associated lymphoid system (MALT). The disturbance of the associated lymphoid tissue of the digestive mucosa (GALT), due to intestinal dysbiosis, was also reflected in the associated lymphoid tissue of the respiratory mucosa (BALT), in the form of rhinitis and allergic asthma, and in the lymphoid tissue associated urinary mucosa, which was expressed as a recurrent urinary infection. By treating the root of the original disturbance, the GALT digestive system, correcting the intestinal dysbiosis, little by little the entire lymphoid system of all the mucous membranes returned to normal and within nine months, the patient had improved significantly, both of digestive and extra-digestive symptoms, thereby improving her quality of life.

Discussion

This patient's case is an example of the hundreds of thousands of patients who, like her, live on pilgrimages through multiple medical offices of different specialties, in search of a solution for the endless chain of symptoms and problems they suffer.

Lacking the integrative approach, each specialist was limited to treating the disturbed organ for which the patient consulted and thus had treatment for rhinitis and asthma recommended by the allergist, for migraine, recommended by the neurologist, for infection recurrent urinary tract, recommended by the urologist, for irritable colon, recommended by the digestive system; However, since none of these doctors could understand what was really happening with this patient, by not being able to see her as an integrated entity, none of these treatments were satisfactory, and on the contrary, they were more harmful.

In the end, faced with the impotence of being able to solve her chain of health problems, her digestive doctor considered that it was a psychiatric case and chose to refer her to a psychiatrist, so that he could add her cocktail of psychotropic drugs to all the treatments she already had received and surely, they would have contributed to further deteriorating the quality of life of this patient.

The saddest thing that we can highlight in this whole panorama of events that this patient brings us is that none of her treating specialist doctors would have been able to reach the logical and real conclusion that explained the chain of pathophysiological events that arose in her and discover the true actors causing their evils, due to the following reasons:

Most conventional doctors, regardless of their specialty, including gastroenterologists, do not believe in the phenomenon of *food intolerances,* they disqualify and discredit the tests to diagnose them, they even mock and laugh at patients who undergo these tests, which for them have no value.

b.-Everything related to the *Microbiota* suffers the same fate, there are even doctors who do not even know what the word *Microbiota* means. Likewise, the test to evaluate it, unknown to most conventional doctors, is also the object of disqualification, ridicule and discredit.

c.-It should also be noted that all of these tests mentioned, the one for food intolerance mediated by IgG, the one for microbiota, the breath test with measurement of hydrogen and methane in the exhaled air for the diagnosis of lactose and fructose malabsorption sorbitol, lactulose and bacterial overgrowth (SIBO), are also not available to doctors and patients, because they are not performed by the laboratories of most public hospitals and even many private ones, having to resort to special laboratories or research to be able to carry them out.

Finally, it is interesting to ask:

a.-Why does this phenomenon occur within most hospitals and groups of orthodox doctors, with these issues related to the microbiota, food intolerance and intestinal dysbiosis?

b.-Why do most of the existing laboratories in public hospitals, and many of the private ones, do not have the technology to perform all the tests related to these pathologies, which, on the other hand, are not of great complexity and exorbitantly high cost?

c.-Why are these topics censored, discredited, and disqualified by most conventional doctors and hospitals, when they are part of the scientific medical research of recent decades, enjoy prolific publication in many magazines and websites prestige and are many traditional concepts changing in the understanding of many diseases?

The treatment of all these disturbances of nutrition and digestive physiology that are responsible for a chain of pathological events that torment people who suffer from them, as was the case of Teresa, requires nutritional education and dietary changes adjusted to the intolerance test, use of prebiotics and probiotics to correct intestinal dysbiosis, specific use of supplements such as glutamine, zinc, vitamin A and D to improve intestinal barrier function.

Since none of these therapeutic elements can be synthesized in a capsule or tablet, sold in pharmacies, and fill the coffers of the pharmaceutical chemical industry, this is most likely where the answer to our questions lies. Simply put, all medical knowledge that is not highly profitable for the pharmaceutical chemical industry is disqualified, discredited, and labeled unscientific.

As this industry exercises an almost hypnotic and sacrosanct power over most conventional doctors, they simply follow the guidelines set forth by this industry and act in accordance with the paradigms created by it, and the most dramatic thing is that most of these good doctors are not even aware of this reality.

Chapter 4

Peter feels very exhausted

In June 2017, Peter, a 26-year-old man, began to worry about his health because he had been feeling a sensation of erectile dysfunction for weeks and his partner was already noticing it. He also realized that for the same time he had been experiencing a strange, permanent, irrecoverable tiredness even if he slept well at night or took a nap during the day, then, a few months later, a lack of concentration appeared, a permanent feeling of cold in everything. the body and skin very dry.

In January 2018, Peter was alarmed by his difficulty in erection and decided to consult his primary care doctor, who, after performing some laboratory tests and observing an altered thyroid value, decided to send him to an Endocrinologist. The endocrine doctor repeated the tests and confirmed an elevated TSH (thyrotropin hormone) value, it was 7.2 mg, with the normal range being between 0.8 to 5 mg. With this result he told Peter that he had a disease called *Hypothyroidism*, which was the explanation for all the symptoms that he had been having for 8 months.

Peter was alarmed when he heard what the endocrine doctor told him and asked him if he had any solution or if it was a lifelong illness, in addition to the long-term consequences, because he was very young. He also asked if further tests were necessary to investigate the cause of this disease.

The endocrine doctor responded that this disease was very common in women but could also affect men at any age, that the cause was unknown and was usually due to an immunological disorder that had no cure. He told him that he would have to take a medication called

Eutirox for the rest of his life, which was thyroid hormone replacement, because his diseased thyroid gland could not produce that hormone normally and insisted that he start treatment as soon as possible to avoid the possible complications that could arise, such as cardiovascular disorders, anemia, fluid retention and infertility. Peter started *Eutirox* that same day and observed that all his symptoms worsened intensely in that first week of treatment, which is why he decided to stop it at his own risk.

Peter came to my office in August 2018, and after telling his story he said that he had three main concerns or doubts:

1.-His endocrine doctor did not show interest in investigating the cause of the hypothyroidism he was complaining about and suggested hormone replacement treatment from the outset, to correct the symptoms, and he was plagued with doubts as to whether the origin of the problem was known and whether it would be corrected, it is likely that the hypothyroidism disappeared.

2.-When starting to take *Eutirox*, he observed a worsening of the symptoms he was experiencing, greater fatigue, weakness, lack of concentration and some insomnia. For this reason, he decided to stop taking it and look for another form of treatment for his disease.

3.-Peter wanted to investigate his health problem from another perspective that did not involve taking *Eutirox* to treat hypothyroidism only symptomatically, and for an indefinite period, and in addition, he was distressed by the side effects of this medication.

What does Conventional Medicine think?

The most common cause of Hypothyroidism, in both men and women, is usually an inflammation of the thyroid gland, known as *Thyroiditis*, which includes a group of individual disorders that inflame the gland and produce a variety of symptoms. For example, *Hashimoto's Thyroiditis* is the most common type of thyroiditis and often presents with symptoms of hypothyroidism, *Puerperal Thyroiditis* is a common cause of hypothyroidism after childbirth, *Subacute Thyroiditis* is the most common cause of pain in the anterior face of the neck, in the area of the thyroid gland and *Thyroiditis medication* is a side effect of some drugs, such as amiodarone (an antiarrhythmic for the heart) and interferon (hepatitis C treatment).

Hashimoto's Thyroiditis, also known as *Chronic Lymphocytic Thyroiditis*, is an autoimmune disorder, in which antibodies directed against the thyroid gland lead to chronic inflammation. It is not known why some people produce these antibodies, although this condition tends to run in families. Over time, however, this leads to a reduced ability of the thyroid gland to produce thyroid hormones, leading to gradual failure and eventually an underactive thyroid, known as Hypothyroidism.

Hashimoto's Thyroiditis occurs most frequently in middle-aged women but can be seen at any age and can also affect men and children.

There are no signs or symptoms that are specific to *Hashimoto's Thyroiditis*. Because the condition usually progresses very slowly over many years, people may not show any symptoms at first, even though typical antibodies against *Thyroperoxidase* (TPO) can be detected in blood tests. However, over time, thyroiditis causes slow, chronic cell damage, leading to the development of a goiter (an enlarged thyroid) with gradual thyroid failure. Eventually, most patients will develop symptoms of hypothyroidism which may include fatigue, weight gain, constipation, increased sensitivity to cold, dry skin, depression, muscle aches and exercise tolerance that is reduced, as well as irregular and heavy menstruation, and erectile dysfunction.

The diagnosis of *Hashimoto's Thyroiditis* is usually made when patients present with symptoms of hypothyroidism, usually accompanied by the presence of a goiter (enlarged thyroid gland) on physical examination, and laboratory tests consistent with hypothyroidism with an elevated level of thyroid TSH in the blood and low levels of thyroid hormone T3 and T4. When measured, levels of thyroid antibodies, called TPO, are usually elevated. TPO is an enzyme that plays an important role in the production of thyroid hormones. Occasionally, the disease can be diagnosed early, especially in people with a strong family history of thyroid disease, or during routine laboratory tests, even before the patient develops symptoms of hypothyroidism.

In these cases, a slight and isolated elevation of TSH in the blood is usually seen, with normal levels of thyroid hormones and positive TPO antibodies.

Patients with elevated TPO antibodies but normal thyroid function tests, TSH, T3, and T4 do not require treatment. For those patients with symptoms of hypothyroidism and elevated TSH with low levels of T3 and T4, treatment consists of thyroid hormone replacement, which, taken orally in an appropriate dose, is inexpensive, very effective in restoring normal hormone levels thyroid and results in an improvement in the symptoms of hypothyroidism. All patients with *Hashimoto's Thyroiditis* who develop hypothyroidism will need lifelong treatment with Levothyroxine (*Eutirox*).

What does non-conventional medicine think?

Most doctors know that hypothyroidism is an autoimmune disease, but most patients don't know it. The reason doctors don't tell their patients is simple: it doesn't affect their treatment plan. Conventional medicine does not have effective treatments for autoimmune diseases; they typically use corticosteroids and other medications to suppress the immune system in certain conditions, such as multiple sclerosis, rheumatoid arthritis, and Crohn's disease, with often potentially more harmful effects.

But in the case of *Hashimoto*, it is believed that the consequences, that is, the side effects and complications of using immunosuppressive medications, outweigh the potential benefits.

So, the standard procedure for a *Hashimoto's* patient is to simply wait until the immune system has destroyed enough thyroid tissue and then give them thyroid hormone replacement. If other commonly associated symptoms begin to occur, such as depression or insulin resistance, additional medications are prescribed for these problems, such as metformin. The obvious shortcoming of this approach is that it does not treat the underlying cause of the problem, which is the immune system attacking the thyroid gland, and if the underlying cause is not treated, the treatment is not going to work very well.

Hashimoto's disease often manifests as a poly-endocrine autoimmune pattern. This means that in addition to having antibodies against thyroid tissue, it is not uncommon for *Hashimoto's* patients to also have antibodies against other tissues or enzymes. The most common are transglutaminase (celiac disease), cerebellum (neurological disorders), intrinsic factor (pernicious anemia), glutamic acid decarboxylase (anxiety/panic attacks), and late-onset type 1 diabetes. What most patients with hypothyroidism need to understand is that they do not have a problem with their thyroid, but rather they have a problem with their immune system attacking the thyroid.

Several studies show a strong relationship between autoimmune thyroid disease (both *Hashimoto's and Graves'*) and gluten intolerance. The relationship is so well established that researchers suggest that all people with autoimmune thyroid disease be screened for gluten intolerance, and vice versa.

How is the connection explained? Is it a case of mistaken identity? The molecular structure of gliadin, the protein portion of gluten, closely resembles that of the thyroid gland. When gliadin breaks through the protective barrier of the intestine and enters the bloodstream, the immune system marks it for destruction. These antibodies against gliadin also cause the body, out of confusion, to attack the thyroid tissue, and this is called *molecular mimicry*. Even worse, the immune response to gluten can last up to 6 months each time it is consumed.

One of the reasons why gluten intolerance is almost never detected is that both doctors and patients mistakenly believe that it only causes digestive problems. But gluten intolerance can also present with inflammation in the joints (arthritis), skin (acne), airways (asthma), brain, (neuroinflammation) and thyroid (thyroiditis), and often without obvious symptoms in the intestines.

Foods containing gluten (both whole grains and flours) often also contain substances that inhibit nutrient absorption, damage our intestinal lining, and activate a potentially destructive autoimmune response. Additionally, there are no nutrients in gluten-containing foods that cannot be easily and efficiently obtained from gluten-free foods.

What was the treatment and evolution that Peter followed?

We subjected Peter to a series of tests, both laboratory and thyroid ultrasound, and we observed the following:

a.-His TSH values in September 2018 were still somewhat elevated, 6.6 with a normal value of 5.3. However, all his other thyroid hormone values were within the normal range:

- Total T3 ....1.25 (normal 0.4 to 1.6)
- Free T3 ....3.6 (normal 3 to 8.5)
- Total T4 ....10 (normal 4 to 12)
- Free T4...................... 0.89. (normal 0.5 to 1.4)

b.-An elevation of anti-thyroid antibodies was evident:

- Anti TPO...................962 (normal 0.1 to 5.6)

c.-Sex hormonal tests were also performed, and some alterations were found in his values:

- Prolactin ....32 (normal 2.6 to 13)
- Progesterone.....................1.2 (normal up to 0.6)
- Estradiol......................35 (normal 15 to 33)
- DHEA............................13.9 (normal up to 9)
- Free Testosterone.........13 (normal 4.7 to 24)

d.-Thyroid ultrasound revealed a gland of normal size, homogeneous and without focal lesions.

Given the presence of symptoms of hypothyroidism, with high values of TSH, prolactin and TPO antibodies, we considered the diagnosis of *"Hashimoto's Autoimmune Thyroiditis"* as the basic cause of the thyroid disorder.

The normality of the thyroid ultrasound made us think that the disorder the autoimmune disease was recent and had not yet significantly damaged the thyroid gland, and therefore, a remedial treatment could be attempted in an integrative manner.

Considering that Peter reported in his medical history that he had also been suffering for months from digestive symptoms manifested by heaviness and pain in the stomach after eating, flatulence, gas and abdominal bloating, and he related them to wheat-based foods; We suspect that he might have a *gluten intolerance* and this food intolerance could be the cause of the thyroid problem.

Based on the suspicion that Peter suffered from gluten intolerance, we decided to give him the following treatment:

a.-Eat a 100% gluten-free diet for 3 months

b.-Nutritional supplementation to strengthen the thyroid gland: L-tyrosine, iodine, vitamins, and minerals.

c.-Plants with anti-inflammatory power: Curcuma Longa, Boswellia Serratia, Harpagofito.

d.-Supplements to improve intestinal permeability: vitamin A, D, Zinc, Glutamine.

e.-Prebiotics and Probiotics to improve the intestinal ecosystem

f.-Catalytic oligotherapy to improve the functioning of the Hypothalamus-Pituitary-Thyroid axis.

After the first 3 months of treatment the results obtained were the following:

a.-Complete disappearance of hypothyroidism symptoms

b.-Significant improvement in erectile dysfunction

c.-Normalization of TSH values and anti-TPO antibodies

d.-Normalization of prolactin, estradiol, progesterone, and DHEA values

Peter was followed in consultation for a year and his clinical stability and maintenance of normality in his laboratory tests could be evidenced, and he was discharged from the Endocrinology consultation in July 2019.

Conclusions

1.-Peter consulted for a clinical picture of Hypothyroidism treated with synthetic hormone replacement using the medication *Eutirox*, which caused a worsening of his symptoms.

2.-His endocrine doctor did not perform tests to investigate the cause of hypothyroidism and that made him decide to look for other forms of treatment for his health problem.

3.-Laboratory tests revealed the presence of Anti-TPO type autoantibodies in high values, about two hundred times above their minimum normal value. This made us consider the diagnosis of *Hashimoto's chronic lymphocytic thyroiditis*.

4.-Considering that he also had digestive symptoms related to gluten-based foods, and the relationship between *Hashimoto's Thyroiditis* and gluten intolerance being known and reported in the medical literature, we decided to prescribe a 100% gluten-free diet as a basis. of his treatment.

5.-We complement the treatment based on nutritional supplementation for:
- Nourish and strengthen the thyroid gland
- Reduce inflammation of the thyroid tissue
- Improve the barrier function and ecosystem of the intestine
- Improve the hypothalamic-pituitary-thyroid endocrine axis

6.-The clinical and laboratory results obtained were highly satisfactory for the patient, and one year after completing his integrative treatment he was discharged from the Endocrinology consultation and did not need to continue taking the medication (*Eutirox*) initially indicated.

Discussion

The phrase: "*You suffer from an incurable disease of unknown cause and must take medical treatment for life,*" is something that every student learned in the Faculty of Medicine when he was training as a doctor, because it was very common and recurring for many diseases, such as all *Autoimmune* such as rheumatoid arthritis, lupus erythematosus, ulcerative colitis, psoriasis, etc. It was also the phrase that accompanied *Chronic diseases*, such as diabetes, high blood pressure, atherosclerosis, heart disease, bronchial asthma, etc.

And of course, also for *Degenerative Diseases* such as leukemia, cancer, multiple sclerosis, Alzheimer's, and Parkinson's, to mention the most common.

When we were medical students and we heard that phrase recurrently throughout our entire career, we never questioned it and accepted it as an inexorable truth and like many other truths that were also instilled in us during those 7 years that we were in training. We kept it in our minds, in our medical bag and in the pocket of our white coat, so as not to forget it and then sing it to all those patients who came to our office and were diagnosed with a chronic, degenerative, or autoimmune disease. And so that we would not forget that truth, or so that we would not question it at any time, they continued to repeat and reinforce it to us when we completed the master's degree in medical specialization, and in all the courses, conferences, and update workshops that we held. We continue to do so for the rest of our lives as medical professionals.

Peter's clinical case is proof that this supposed inexorable truth of an incurable disease, of unknown cause and requiring lifelong pharmacological treatment, is, and has always been, false, and in saying so, it may sound surprising, however, it is the truth. After having ventured into the world of Integrative Medicine in the last 20 years, it has been the patients themselves who have shown me this reality, and all the clinical cases that I have presented to them are an example of this.

Now, looking back, I must recognize that this truth that I learned in medical school and repeated for 15 years in more than ten hospitals in which I worked and trained as a specialist in internal medicine and cardiology, was conditioned to the paradigm, methodology and orthodox pharmacological treatment protocols.

Diseases classified by conventional medicine as *incurable* are only so, under the approach and treatment that that medicine applies to them, simply because the reasoning and understanding of the disease is incorrect, and therefore, the result of the treatment applied it is discouraging because it only manages to lessen the symptoms, at best.

It is not that conventional doctors who work in clinics and hospitals where official medicine is practiced are bad doctors, in truth they are not, because they all studied between 6 to 8 years in medical school to obtain their medical degree, many continued studying for another 5 or more years to complete their specialization and as many others to achieve super specialization or doctorate (PHD). A whole path full of struggle, sacrifice, night guards and thousands of hard and difficult experiences that only the pure and true vocation of service can help us tolerate, endure, and even enjoy.

It is simply that all conventional hospital doctors, who are good doctors, are unaware and do not have any information about the other paradigm, that of the other medicine, the so-called *non-conventional*, which enjoys the support of the World Health Organization and is expressed in magazines, associations, organizations, congresses and countless events and institutions of an eminently scientific nature, supported by serious and rigorous research, as valid as that of conventional medicine.

The good endocrine doctor who treated Peter did what he learned, acted based on the knowledge he had and could not do anything else, simply because he had no information that there was anything else.

He was not aware of the relationship that exists between gluten intolerance and *Hashimoto's Thyroiditis*, much less the application of nutritherapy, natural supplementation and medicinal plants to correct this digestive and immune imbalance. If he had known, he would surely have applied that knowledge to help his patient and would have obtained the same favorable results.

It is likely that someone who is reading these reasonings and arguments will wonder why conventional doctors do not have or know the same information that non-conventional doctors handle, if at the end of the day, everything is published and simply by accessing any online search engine they can download that information and find out about the issue and proceed with it.

I was also an orthodox and conventional doctor, pure and simple, during the first 15 years of professional practice, and I was also in those shoes, completely unaware of the world of unconventional medicine. In my humble opinion, based on the experience of having lived within the two medicines, the explanation for this situation that I am arguing lies in the role and manipulation exercised by the omnipresent pharmaceutical chemical industry.

This industry is responsible for keeping conventional doctors hypnotized with all its legal tricks, making them believe that only the research carried out and sponsored by it is truly scientific and supports the inexorable truths of medicine.

Every doctor who feels worthy and respectful of being one must profess and defend these truths.

But the matter does not end there, the omnipotent chemical pharmaceutical industry has also taken it upon itself to discredit, disqualify and excommunicate the entire world of unconventional medicine and all those who believe, participate, and use its knowledge, whom it describes as pseudoscientists and quackery.

To ensure that conventional, orthodox and official doctor, of whom it believes itself to be the owner and mistress, will ever think of snooping, investigating or flirting with the sects that practice other medicine, the multimillion-dollar and all-powerful chemical pharmaceutical industry has assured the support and complicity of medical associations, ministries of health, and even the governments of nations and all the mass media, to accuse, point out, persecute and punish any doctor who tries to change sides .

For all this, the vast majority of conventional doctors echo this giant trap and are not interested in what other medicine may have to say about any medical topic, and if you hear or read something about it, they do not give it any credit. , and if by chance he were to doubt for a moment, only the terror of feeling singled out, questioned and segregated by his conventional medical profession forces him to rule out any possibility of change and ends up silencing his professional and scientific conscience that screams at him from your vocation, what if it's true?.

Chapter 5

Louise can't get pregnant

Luisa is a 29-year-old woman who wanted to get pregnant. She got married at age 27 and for the next 2 years she tried to get pregnant without success. She had her first period at 15 years old and they were always painful. At 18 years old, she was diagnosed with *Endometriosis* in both ovaries and was treated with contraceptives for 8 consecutive years. In October 2016, Luisa went to an Assisted Fertility center with the hope of seeing her dream come true.

At the assisted fertilization center she was diagnosed with low ovarian reserve due to *Endometriosis* that she suffered from. The only solution they offered was *In Vitro Fertilization*. For 3 months she was given injected hormones, then in the ovarian puncture 5 mature eggs were obtained, of which 3 were fertilized in vitro and two of them evolved to become an embryo. Everything had progressed wonderfully and in December 2016 she had her 2 embryos implanted and she was scheduled for an appointment in a month to confirm her pregnancy.

In January 2017, when she was tested for pregnancy, the result was negative. The in vitro fertilization procedure failed in the final phase. The patient and her family were devastated and disappointed, and the question on everyone's mind was why? What had gone wrong if everything seemed to be going correctly? The medical team that treated her simply said: *"that is normal for it to happen, these are the expected statistical probabilities".*

"Some women require several in vitro fertilization procedures to achieve pregnancy, perhaps that is your case."

What does Conventional Medicine think?

Infertility is defined as the attempt to have a child, maintaining frequent sexual relations, for at least one year, without success. This problem affects millions of couples in the world. It is estimated that between 10% and 18% of couples have problems having a baby or achieving a successful birth. There are many treatments available, which will depend on the cause of the infertility. After trying to have a child for two years, around 95 percent of couples successfully conceive, following an assisted fertilization method.

Statistics reveal that the causes of infertility in couples are 30% due to female causes, another 30% to male causes, 20% to a combination of both and the remaining 20% is of unknown origin. When the dominant cause is female, it is usually due to three fundamental factors, endometriosis (30%), lack of ovulation (25%) and low ovarian reserve (20%).

The main symptom of infertility is the inability to get pregnant. A menstrual cycle that is too long (35 days or more), too short (less than 21 days), irregular, or absent may mean no ovulation. There likely will be no other obvious signs or symptoms. When to seek medical help depends on age:

*Up to age 35, doctors recommend trying to get pregnant for at least a year before seeking help.

*If you are between 35 and 40 years old, you should consult your doctor after trying 6 months without success.

*If you are over 40, your doctor may want to start testing or treatment right away.

Your doctor may also want to perform tests or treatments right away if you or your partner has known fertility problems, or if you have a history of pelvic inflammatory disease, repeated miscarriages, cancer treatment, or endometriosis. The female infertility study plan includes a series of tests including:

*-Ovulation check

*-Ovarian reserve analysis

*-Hormonal studies

*-Special tests: Ultrasound, Hysterography, etc.

*-Laparoscopy: to investigate endometriosis or tubal cysts

Treatment of female infertility depends on the cause, age, the amount of time you have been infertile, and personal preferences. Infertility is a complex disorder, so treatment involves significant financial, physical, psychological, and time commitments. Although some women need only one or two treatments to restore fertility, several different types of treatments may be needed. Treatments may attempt to restore fertility through medications or surgery, or help you get pregnant through sophisticated techniques.

Currently there are three ways to treat female infertility, which are:

*-Restore fertility with medications

*-Restore fertility with surgery

*-Assisted fertility techniques

If the infertility problem is due to lack of ovulation, it is treated with medications that stimulate the ovaries to correct this problem. This type of drugs can cause adverse effects that must be considered, such as:

*-Multiple pregnancy: a risk of 10-30%

*-Ovarian hyperstimulation: painful ovulations.

*-Ovarian tumors in the future: if taken for more than 1 year

There are several surgical procedures that can reverse problems or improve female fertility. However, surgical treatments for fertility are not common today due to the success of other treatments.

The most common methods of assisted reproduction include the following:

*Intrauterine insemination (IUI). Millions of healthy sperm are placed inside the uterus, near the time of ovulation.

*In vitro fertilization (IVF). This involves obtaining mature eggs from a woman and fertilizing them with a man's sperm on a plate in a laboratory. The embryos are then transferred to the uterus after

fertilization. IVF is the most effective form of assisted reproductive technology. The IVF cycle takes several weeks and requires regular blood tests and daily hormone injections.

What does non-conventional medicine think?

Fertility, both male and female, is a property linked to the person's state of health and is related to aspects such as weight, nutritional status, certain micronutrients, and the microbiota.

*-Weight and Fertility:

There is a relationship between body weight and fertility, both female and male. Maintaining an adequate weight will influence the chances of pregnancy, and therefore the success of assisted reproduction treatment, if applicable. That is why it is very important to always eat a balanced diet.

Overweight women undergoing in vitro fertilization treatment will need more hormones to stimulate egg production. Increased medication carries a greater risk of suffering side effects, as well as a greater economic cost of treatment.

Likewise, being underweight can also be detrimental to fertility. According to the WHO, a normal weight would be a BMI between 18.5 and 24.9. Therefore, a BMI below 18.5 is considered underweight. It is estimated that the ideal weight when getting pregnant should be a BMI between 20 and 22.

*-Micronutrients and Fertility

There are medical studies that have shown the importance of certain nutrients in fertility, and how low levels of them can significantly affect reproductive capacity.

.-Vitamin D: The association of vitamin D and reproduction derives from several studies in which it has been seen that there is the presence of receptors for this vitamin in many tissues of the reproductive system in both sexes. In 2014, a study was published that demonstrated this, that women with correct levels of this vitamin in their blood had higher implantation percentages.

.-Vitamin B12: It is another of the essential vitamins to improve fertility in both sexes. This vitamin is very important in cell growth, it intervenes in an important way in the synthesis of DNA. But in addition, vitamin B12 also plays an important role in the work carried out by the thyroid and let us remember that the thyroid has to be well regulated so that adequate embryo implantation occurs and that abortions do not occur.

.-Uterine microbiota: More than 166 different genera of bacteria coexist in the uterus, this is what we call the uterine microbiota. According to a study published in the *American Journal of Obstetrics and Gynecology* in December 2016, the bacterial flora of the uterus influences the success of pregnancy. This will allow probiotic treatment to be administered to the uterine cavity, if bacteria of the *Lactobacillus* genus do not dominate, before the transfer of the embryos. This will increase the chances of the embryo implanting and the pregnancy reaching term, without an abortion occurring for this reason.

*-Acupuncture and Fertility

Chinese medicine has had treatments for female fertility for more than a thousand years and has had a Gynecological specialty for more than 700. Due to the benefits that acupuncture brings to fertility, many assisted reproduction clinics already include a specialized unit for this millennial technique. The British Medical Journal has recently published an analysis that compiles all the data from recent research on the effects of acupuncture on in vitro fertility cycles. The study showed a 65% increase in pregnancy establishment, an 87% increase in pregnancy continuity and a 91% increase in live births.

What was the treatment that Luisa followed?

The initial clinical evaluation that we performed on Luisa in March 2018 revealed some additional alterations, which in summary were the following:

*She suffered from monthly migraines since she was 24 years old, which she treated with paracetamol.

*She suffered from chronic tonsillitis with 6 episodes per year that were treated with antibiotics.

*She also suffered from repetitive urinary tract infections of up to 3 attacks per year, which she also treated with antibiotics.

* She had digestive disorders since adolescence with dyspepsia, constipation, and internal hemorrhoids.

* Her diet was highly acidifying and pro-inflammatory with excess animal products, red meat, sausages, cow's milk and dairy derivatives, refined flours and various sweets, and an addiction to chocolate.

* The physical examination revealed signs of poor nutrition and nutritional deficiencies, she was pale and had a body mass index (BMI) of 14.6.

* In addition, hypertrophic tonsils with crypts were seen, and all her bones were painful to manual pressure.

*Pelvic ultrasound demonstrated the presence of endometriotic cysts in both ovaries.

*Laboratory tests also reflected some alterations:

- Anemia with hemoglobin of 11 gr/dl (normal 12 to 15 gr/dl)
- Low cholesterol: 130 mg/dl (normal value 160 to 220 mg/dl)
- Low vitamin B12: 175 mg/dl. (normal 250 to 950mg/dl)
- Low vitamin D: 28 pgr/ml (normal 30 to 90 pgr/ml)
- Low ovarian anti-Mullerian: 1.89 (normal value 6-9 ngr/ml)

We consider that to achieve an effective result in a second in vitro fertilization, Luisa should receive an integrative treatment for:

.-Improve her nutritional level, recover her ideal weight and overcome all nutritional deficiencies observed.

.-Correct the other health disorders that she accused: chronic pharyngitis, digestive disorders, migraines and urinary infections.

.-Normalize her anti-Mullerian hormonal values to increase the possibility of pregnancy.

With this working hypothesis we designed a treatment scheme that the patient followed for 9 months, which consisted of:

.-Nutritional evaluation and control to follow an alkaline, high-protein diet, low in gluten and other pro-inflammatory elements.

.-Nutritional supplementation with multivitamins, multimineral, multi aminoacids, omega 3-6-9 fatty acids, vitamin D3 (5000 IU daily) and intramuscular group B vitamin complex until B12 values normalize and then we move on to oral maintenance.

.-Acupuncture in weekly sessions for 1 month and then biweekly for 7 months to stimulate ovarian function and promote follicular development.

How was Luisa's clinical evolution?

Luisa completed all the treatment rigorously and attended her medical check-ups every 3 months to verify the nutritional recovery sought. After 9 months of treatment, her laboratory analysis reflected better values:

- Hemoglobin of 13.5 g,
- Total cholesterol 165 mg,
- Vitamin B12: 760 mg, Vitamin D: 70 ngr
- All sex hormones were in normal values
- Anti-Mullerian hormone rose to 5 ngr/ml

The patient gained weight and her BMI rose to 18.0. She remained free of tonsillitis, migraines, and urinary tract infection during the 9 months of treatment.

In December 2017, the patient decided to undergo a second assisted fertilization, achieving the maturation of several follicles to an advanced level, 8 mature eggs were obtained, and 5 eggs were fertilized in vitro. The patient decided to implant two fertile eggs and the other 3 fertilized eggs were frozen. In January 2018 it was confirmed that Luisa had become pregnant and 9 months later a healthy girl was born.

Conclusion and Discussion

This clinical case of female infertility shows us how *integrative medicine* works and the results that can be obtained when doctor and patient work as a team, each fulfilling their corresponding role in the process.

Luisa had been trying to get pregnant for 2 years without success. She went to an assisted fertilization center and underwent an in vitro fertilization process in December 2016. Although the technical in vitro fertilization procedure was successful and several eggs were fertilized, when they were implanted in the patient's uterus, they did not pregnancy was achieved.

It is highly striking, and criticizable, that the medical team specialized in assisted fertilization did not realize that Luisa, who was going to have a fertilized egg implanted, did not have the most favorable health conditions to guarantee a satisfactory result.

All the medical literature published on this topic insists on the need for every woman who has fertility problems and is going to undergo an assisted fertility process, should receive comprehensive medical care to correct all the alterations that have been detected, both in his laboratory analyzes and in the functioning of all his organs. The uterus where a fertilized egg is going to be implanted is not an organ that lives and functions separately from the female human body, and on the contrary, is in close coexistence with the rest of the organs and with all the biochemistry and physiology of the body organism.

Having overlooked this holistic reality, under which our body functions, must have had a definitive weight that led to the failure of in vitro fertilization in December 2016; and the proof of this is in what happened when after 9 months of an integrative treatment, with the correction of all the nutritional deficiencies found, including low weight, the patient became pregnant after undergoing a second in vitro fertilization procedure, in December 2017, being able to sustain the pregnancy until the end and end with a normal delivery.

Luisa's experience invites us to make some reflections:

How many patients who undergo an assisted fertilization procedure have lived, are living, or are going to live an experience similar to Luisa's?

How much frustration, disappointment, and suffering could we save patients if we saw them as human beings whose bodies function as an integrated whole?

How much good would we do for humanity if we were the doctors it needs, with a holistic vision of the human being, with an ecological approach to the environment, respecting the ancient heritage of the great doctors of the golden past of vitalist medicine and complying with a professional exercise framed in deontology and ethics?.

Chapter 6

Mary is vomiting blood.

Mary is a 43-year-old woman, a hotel receptionist, who presented, on the night of July 9, 2016, intense abdominal pain accompanied by nausea, vomiting blood, and great general weakness. Her family took her to the emergency room where she was hospitalized. The first laboratory tests that were performed revealed that she had intense anemia, with a hemoglobin value of 5 grams (normal 12 to 14 grams), she also had very low red blood cells, at 1.2 million/ml (normal 3.5 to 5 million/ml), white blood cells, at 3000/ml (normal 4.5 to 10,000/ml) and platelets, at 44,000/ml (normal 150 thousand to 450 thousand/ml). In view of these results, she was evaluated by a Hematologist who ordered blood transfusions and said that she should rule out leukemia.

Fortunately, Mary managed to stabilize in the first 24 hours, after having received 2 blood transfusions and intravenous medication. The doctor decided to discharge her to her home with oral medication and gave her an appointment at the Hematology Service for her to come in a month and begin studies to clarify the suspicion of leukemia.

Mary visited me five days after leaving the hospital and she was apprehensive and afraid that she might have leukemia, with the possibility of having to undergo chemotherapy treatment. She hoped to find another solution, one that would offer a different expectation than what conventional medicine had offered her.

What does Conventional Medicine think?

There is a medical condition called Medullary Aplasia or Aplastic Anemia, a disease that belongs to the failure syndrome of the bone marrow (place where blood cells are made), characterized by a significant reduction in the three types of cells that circulate in the blood, erythrocytes, leukocytes, and platelets, which is known as Pancytopenia.

The incidence of Aplastic Anemia is 0.6 to 6.1 cases per million inhabitants and usually appears at three times in life, the first peak occurs in childhood, between 2 and 5 years, a more common peak occurs between 15 and 30 years, and another after 55 years. Depending on the cause there are two types, acquired (80%) and hereditary (20%). Between 65 and 70% of cases of acquired medullary aplasia (MA) have an unknown cause (idiopathic), 25% are due to medications and less than 5% are due to a viral infection.

In medullary aplasia, because of the lack of blood cell production, patients may present different symptoms to a variable degree depending on the intensity of the deficit. A deficiency of red blood cells (anemia) can manifest itself with fatigue, weakness, paleness, a feeling of dizziness, palpitations, and headache. Because of the deficiency in white blood cells (leukopenia), mouth ulcers and infections can occur on a continuous basis. A deficiency in platelets (thrombopenia) can cause bruising after minimal trauma, bleeding from the gums, nose, or conjunctivae, as well as more serious bleeding elsewhere in the body.

The diagnosis of aplastic anemia is usually made with two types of tests:

*-Blood analysis: to detect the decrease in all blood cells (pancytopenia).

*-Bone marrow biopsy: it is the confirmatory test. A doctor uses a needle to remove a small sample of bone marrow from a large bone in the body, such as the hip bone. In aplastic anemia, the bone marrow contains fewer blood cells than normal.

Treatments for aplastic anemia, which will depend on the severity of your condition and your age, may include observation, blood transfusions, medications, or a bone marrow transplant. Severe aplastic anemia, in which the blood cell count is extremely low, is life-threatening and requires immediate hospitalization.

Aplastic anemia caused by drugs, such as that which occurs during cancer chemotherapy, usually improves when the medication is stopped. There is also aplastic anemia related to pregnancy, which usually improves once it ends. In any case, if aplastic anemia persists after the medication or pregnancy disappears, specific treatment must be started.

What does non-conventional medicine think?

There are a series of risk factors that can increase the chances of a person suffering from aplastic anemia, the most common being the following:

*-Chemo and radiotherapy against cancer

   *-Exposure to toxic substances such as pesticides and solvents

   *-Certain commonly used medications

   *-Blood diseases, autoimmunity, and serious infections

   *-In rare cases, pregnancy.

When a person is exposed to these risk factors, they should be very vigilant for possible symptoms of possible pancytopenia and ask their doctor to perform blood tests to monitor their blood cell count.

Once you are diagnosed with aplastic anemia, it is advisable to follow the following advice:

   *-Stop any medication you may be taking that may be the cause of aplastic anemia.

   *-Make changes to your diet and take mineral and vitamin supplements to provide enough nutrients to your bone marrow to help it make blood cells.

   *-Take preventive measures to help tolerate symptoms and prevent problems caused by pancytopenia.

- Rest to compensate for fatigue due to anemia
- Avoid trauma that could cause bleeding
- Protect yourself from germs

*-Work with your doctor to investigate and correct the possible cause that is generating spinal aplasia.

What was the treatment followed by Mary?

When taking Mary's clinical history, there was a piece of information of great interest. She had been diagnosed at 23 years of age with *Rheumatoid Polyarthritis* due to generalized joint pain that she suffered cyclically coinciding with the winter seasons; Due to this, she attended a *Rheumatology* consultation and was medicated with *Hydroxychloroquine*, which she had been consuming for 10 years. It turns out that one of the side effects of this medication is that it can cause pancytopenia due to spinal aplasia, as Mary had suffered.

It was logical to hypothesize that Mary had presented with aplastic anemia secondary to the toxic action of *Hydroxychloroquine*, which she had been taking for 10 years. Based on this hypothesis, we indicate the following treatment scheme:

a.-Immediate and definitive suspension of *Hydroxychloroquine*

b.-Gastric protection diet with prebiotics, probiotics, and glutamine, to avoid other digestive bleeding.

c.-Supplementation with multivitamins and multiminerals

d.-Hematin supplementation based on highly concentrated oral iron associated with group B vitamins and vitamin C to improve its absorption.

e.-Medicinal mushrooms such as Reishi, Maitake, Shiitake, Turkey Tail and Cordyceps as immunostimulants.

f.-Shark liver oil, rich in Alkylglycerol, a compound that stimulates the production of white blood cells in the bone marrow.

How did Mary evolve with the indicated treatment?

Two months after having suspended hydroxychloroquine and undergoing recovery treatment based on nutrition and supplementation, Mary had improved all her symptoms:

*-Hemorrhagic phenomena, such as bleeding gums and vomiting blood, disappeared.

*-She improved symptoms of anemia, paleness, physical and mental fatigue

* -Her laboratory tests were corrected: hemoglobin rose to 14 grams, erythrocytes to 4.5 million, leukocytes to 6000 and platelets reached 282 thousand. The Pancytopenia had resolved.

*-The hematologist ruled out the need to perform a bone marrow puncture after verifying both the improvement in symptoms and the normalization of laboratory results.

Six months later, Mary continued to show clinical improvement, she had not had any episode of oral or digestive bleeding and all symptoms of anemia had disappeared. She was discharged from the hematology service and did not require any special treatment or procedure.

Mary was followed in the Integrative Medicine consultation for 3 years, until July 2019, when she was discharged and maintained the clinical and laboratory normality achieved from the beginning with the indicated treatment.

Conclusion and Discussion

Mary's story is a typical case of medical *iatrogenesis*. The word *iatrogenic* has the literal meaning *"caused by the doctor or healer"*. It is an unwanted or unsought harm to health, caused or provoked, as an inevitable side effect, by a legitimate and endorsed medical act, intended to cure, or improve a specific pathology.

There are several causes of iatrogenesis:

• Medical error

• Medical negligence or improper procedures

• Errors when writing the recipe or recipe that is difficult to decipher.

- Prescription drug interaction.
- Adverse effects of prescribed medications.
- Do not consider the negative effects of the medication
- Overuse of antibiotics leading to resistance
- Unsafe treatments
- Misdiagnosis
- Ignore the negative effects that a medication produces.
- Nosocomial or hospital-acquired infections

In a study published in the journal JAMA in December 1999 by Dr. Bárbara Starfield, from the John Hopkins School of Hygiene and Public Health and based on data that come from studies carried out on hospitalized patients, it reflected conclusive figures of deaths due to medical iatrogenesis. 250,000 deaths were recorded per year, making it the third leading cause of death in the US, after cardiovascular disease and cancer.

The analysis of those 250,000 deaths caused by medical iatrogenesis showed the following causes:
- 12,000 for unnecessary surgeries
- 8,000 due to medication errors in hospitals
- 20,000 for other errors in hospitals
- 80,000 due to infections contracted in hospitals
- 130,000 for negative side effects of medications

Mary's case meets all the conditions to be classified as medical iatrogenesis, and it almost cost her life. There was iatrogenesis in several phases of its history:

* -When her Rheumatologist recommended *Hydroxychloroquine* to treat Rheumatoid Arthritis for a long time, without routine and rigorous laboratory controls to detect possible side effects that would require reducing the dose or discontinuing the medication.

*-When the doctor on duty who received her in the emergency room on the night of July 9, 2016, with digestive bleeding, did not realize that the patient was taking hydroxychloroquine for a long time, a medication that can produce a clinical picture of medullary aplasia as a side effect.

*-When the hematologist who evaluated her that night, he also did not realize that the patient was taking hydroxychloroquine and therefore, the possibility of iatrogenic medullary aplasia was not considered as the cause of all the symptoms that led her to the hospital emergency room

* -When the patient was discharged from a medical emergency and was told to continue taking the hydroxychloroquine prescribed by the Rheumatologist for the treatment of Rheumatoid Arthritis.

The Side Effects of pharmaceutical medications represent one of the main Achilles heels of conventional medicine, because it contradicts the first Hippocratic principle of medicine, *"First do no harm"*, and is also one of the main reasons why many patients every day consider seeking a less harmful medical solution to treat their health problems.

Most orthodox doctors do not worry about making sure that their patient could develop a side effect with the medication they are prescribing, in fact, many of them tell their patients *"do not read the package inserts for the medications I am giving you"* ; nor does it make an effort to monitor the medication that the patient takes for a long time, in order to detect the right moment at which the dose should be lowered, suspended or changed, to avoid possible side effects that can deteriorate the patient's quality of life or worse, threaten their life, as happened with Mary.

In the opinion of many doctors, the increasing refinement of official medicine makes it inevitable that the frequency of iatrogenic diseases will increase every day. However, the risks can be reduced by improving the training of doctors and regular monitoring of their practice in all health institutions. On the other hand, the experimentation to which commercial drugs are subjected before putting them on sale should be exhaustive, to reduce the probability of producing unexpected reactions, and the ministries of health of all nations should ensure compliance with this regulation, which unfortunately, today, is increasingly questioned.

Chapter 7

Ramon has a Crooked Face

Ramón, a 46-year-old man, woke up on the morning of May 12, 2018 with something strange on his face, his right eye was burning, he could hardly close it and it was watering, his mouth was deviated to the left, he could hardly speak and the water fell when he drank it, when he looked in the mirror he realized that he had a very strange expression, because half his face was paralyzed. He felt panic, he thought that it could be irreversible and permanent and that he could also lose his job, which is public facing.

Ramón immediately went to the emergency room where a Neurologist examined him and told him that he had *"Peripheral Facial Paralysis."* To his surprise, they did not prescribe any treatment and only told him to make an appointment with his primary care doctor, who saw him 5 days later to refer him to physical therapy and to be evaluated by an ENT doctor. The appointment for both references was given for 45 days later, and he had to wait that time, without receiving any kind of treatment.

The reality for Ramón is that he had half his face paralyzed and had to wait 45 days to be treated by specialist doctors who would indicate a treatment to recover from his disorder and meanwhile he had to wait all that time without any treatment.

Ramón did a search on the internet and there were two points that worried him:

1.-The importance of starting treatment within the first 72 hours of facial paralysis, to have a greater chance of recovering normality in the shortest time possible.

2.-Some cases may take 3 to 6 months to recover, and worse still, there is the possibility that the symptoms do not disappear completely and last indefinitely.

For these reasons he decided to look for a different option than the one offered by the official health system.

What does Conventional Medicine think?

Idiopathic or primary peripheral facial paralysis is one that has an acute onset and has no known cause. In the past it was associated with sudden cooling of the face (paralysis a frigore), however, currently the etiology is attributed to an inflammatory process in the nerve due to a viral infection (herpes virus). It is unilateral in 99% of cases. It causes paralysis of the muscles innervated by the temporofacial and cervicofacial branches of the facial nerve, causing total or partial loss of voluntary, reflex, and automatic movements of these muscles. On the affected side, there is:

- Flattening of frontal wrinkles,
- Lowering of the eyebrow,
- Inability to occlude the eyelid,
- With epiphora or tearing.
- When the patient is asked to close his eyes, the eyeball on the paralyzed side is directed upward.
- The nasolabial fold is effaced, with deviation of the oral commissure to the opposite side.

Other symptoms may include:
- Pain around the jaw and behind the ear
- Ringing in one or both ears,
- Headache and dizziness
- Loss of taste,
- Very sensitive to sound on the affected side
- Speech impairment,
- Difficulty eating or drinking.

Most often these symptoms, which usually begin suddenly and peak within 48 hours, lead to significant facial distortion. Normally mild cases of Bell's palsy disappear within a month, recovery from more severe cases involving total paralysis is variable.

Complications may include:

• Irreversible damage to the facial nerve

• Abnormal new growth of nerve fibers that causes involuntary contraction of certain muscles when trying to move others (synkinesis),

• For example, when you smile, your eye on the affected side may close

• Partial or total blindness of the eye that does not close due to excessive dryness and scratching of the clear protective layer that covers the eye (cornea).

There are no specific tests for Bell's palsy. The doctor will check your face and ask you to move your facial muscles by closing your eyes, raising your eyebrows, showing your teeth, and frowning, among other movements.

Other diseases, such as stroke, infections, Lyme disease, and tumors, can also cause muscle weakness, which can be confused with Bell's palsy. If the source of your symptoms is unclear, your doctor may recommend other tests, such as:

*-Electromyography (EMG). This test can confirm the presence of nerve injury and determine its severity. EMG measures the electrical activity of a muscle in response to a stimulus and the nature and speed of conduction of electrical impulses along the nerve.

*-Diagnostic imaging scans. Sometimes, it will be necessary to perform a magnetic resonance imaging (MRI) or computed tomography (CT) to rule out other possible sources of pressure on the facial nerves, such as tumors or skull fractures.

There is no cure or standard course of treatment for primary peripheral facial paralysis, the most important factor in treatment is eliminating the source of the nerve damage. It is also important to start treatment in the first 72 hours when indicated.

Treatment is divided into two important aspects, medication, and rehabilitation. The prognosis for individuals with primary peripheral facial palsy is generally very good, the extent of nerve damage determines the extent of recovery, improvement is gradual, and recovery times vary. Most recover completely, returning to normal function within 3 to 6 months. For some, however, symptoms may last longer. In some cases, symptoms may never completely go away.

What does non-conventional medicine think?

a.-Food and Supplementation:

One of the therapeutic measures, when you have the disease, is to use large doses of vitamin B12, B6 and Zinc. Various studies point out the benefits of this vitamin therapy, which can help nerve growth. Specialists recommend taking them orally or better yet injecting them.

Other measures that can help may be to eat healthily with fresh vegetables and fruits, avoiding red meat, flour, and gluten. Selenium and magnesium also help the immune system.

b.-Physiotherapy to stimulate the facial nerve and help maintain muscle tone may be beneficial for some people. Massage and facial exercises can help prevent permanent contractures of paralyzed muscles before recovery occurs. Moist heat applied to the affected side of the face can help decrease pain.

c.-Acupuncture is a measure that can be of great help to accelerate the recovery of facial paralysis, serving as a complement to pharmacological treatment. If it is started within the first two weeks of the onset of symptoms, it helps to restore the sensitivity and function of the affected muscles. Acupuncture enhances blood flow in facial microcirculation, which we already know is decreased in facial paralysis. Some studies suggest that acupuncture produces changes in the functional connectivity of the brain, specifically in the primary somatosensory area, which varies depending on the evolutionary stage of the disease.

What was the treatment that Ramón received?

Ramón consulted me on May 17, 2018, and we immediately began the treatment of his pathology based on 3 crucial aspects.

a.-Fight against the possible inflammation that the facial nerve may suffer, using a short course of corticosteroids, since recent studies have shown that *Prednisone* is an effective treatment for Bell's palsy, it reduces inflammation and swelling, and may be effective in improving facial function by limiting or reducing nerve damage.

b.-Provide specific nutrients to promote the recovery of the damage suffered by the myelin sheath and the nerve fibers of the affected facial nerve. We use vitamin B6, B12, Zinc and Glutathione intravenously.

c.-Stimulation of the affected facial nerve with Acupuncture, applying 3 sessions per week to achieve a faster effect and promote recovery of its functions in the shortest possible time.

What evolution did Ramón have?

From the first day of treatment Ramón noticed improvement in the clinical symptoms, especially in the dryness of the right eye and the closing of the upper eyelid.

After a week he had already improved by 50% and after 2 weeks, a 100% recovery was achieved with complete disappearance of all symptoms and complete restoration of the mobility of the muscles of the right side of the face.

When the 45 days were up and Ramón attended the ENT and physiotherapy consultations that were assigned to him by the conventional Social Security Medical Service, there was no longer any sign of facial paralysis, and he was discharged because he no longer needed any treatment.

Ramón was followed up with quarterly consultations for 20 months after his complete recovery and the persistence of normality was confirmed until the time of discharge in January 2020.

Conclusion and Discussion

The medical experience lived by Ramón allows us to highlight three important aspects:

1.-The medical *indolence* that Ramón had to face when he sought refuge in Conventional Medicine to obtain the necessary help to overcome his sudden health problem that subjected him to a few days of anguish, fear, and uncertainty, due to the uncertain prognosis of the same. The Dictionary defines indolence as: "*The inability to be moved or feel affected by something. Laziness, apathy, and insensitivity, especially to pain.*"

The general population asks:

a.-How is it possible that the feeling of indolence has taken root in the institutions that provide medical care?

b.-Isn't this feeling of indolence contradictory to the sacred professional mission of the doctor?

c.-Does not indolence represent a denial of the doctor's vocation?

d.-What hope is left for patients who find themselves with a doctor who treats them with indolence?

e.-Why has the essence of compassion, commitment and dedication been lost in medical practice today?

One might ask: What would have been the evolution and prognosis of the facial paralysis that Ramón suffered if he had followed the guidelines recommended by the doctors who treated him at Social Security?

2.-The high effectiveness demonstrated by the integration of all treatments provided, both conventional and non-conventional, both well documented by medical literature. Ramón obtained a 100% recovery of his symptoms and the complete disappearance of facial paralysis in just 2 weeks, with the application of an integrative treatment.

3.-When checking the good clinical results achieved in Ramón's case, three concerns arise:

a.-Why can Official Medicine not allow itself the possibility of treating patients with primary facial paralysis with a scheme like the one we used with Ramón?

b.-Why is Conventional Medicine not open to the possibility of applying non-conventional therapies supported by scientific studies that demonstrate their effectiveness in the treatment of many diseases, in a kind of *integration* of these therapies with conventional therapies, always looking for the best response from the patient?

c.-What is happening with Medicine? Why has it distanced itself from its fundamental objective, which is to help recover the health of patients, whenever possible, and using all therapies based on scientific evidence?

Chapter 8

Philip has a tumor in his colon.

Philip, a 51-year-old man, was forced to go to the emergency room on the night of December 27, 2017, due to abdominal pain that he had been experiencing for 2 days, which was accompanied by several vomiting and some fever. In the emergency room they performed several tests and concluded that he had Acute Appendicitis, and they sent him to surgery immediately.

When the surgeon opened Philip's abdomen he was surprised, because instead of appendicitis, he found a 7cm tumor located in the right colon, which had the appearance of being malignant. The surgeon removed the entire right colon (hemicolectomy) and several suspicious lymph nodes. The microscope study revealed that it was Colon Cancer, and two of the removed lymph nodes also came out positive for cancer.

A few days later, Felipe had a CT scan of his entire body to investigate whether there was spread of the tumor to other organs, and only two small metastases were found in the liver. For this reason, they planned chemotherapy treatment for him starting in February 2018. They told him that the cancer he suffered was in an advanced state (grade 4) because it had already spread to the lymph nodes and liver, and that the possibility of survival after one year it was low, despite the treatment.

Philip came to my office in January 2018 and after telling his story, he stated that he wanted to receive complementary treatment with two precise objectives:

1.-Increase the chances of success of the cancer eradication treatment, which was about to be received, based on chemotherapy.

2.-Better tolerate the side effects of chemotherapy.

What does Conventional Medicine think?

Colon cancer usually affects older adults, although it can occur at any age. It usually starts as small, benign clumps of cells called polyps that form inside the colon, and over time, some of those polyps can turn into cancer.

Generally, colon cancer begins when healthy cells in the colon develop changes or mutations in their DNA. As the cells accumulate, they form a tumor and over time, the cancer cells can grow to invade and destroy nearby normal tissue and can move to other parts of the body to form deposits there, called metastasis. .

There are some Risk Factors that increase the possibility of someone developing colon cancer, these are:

*-Be over 60 years of age

*-Consume red meats and sausages excessively

*-Have a family history of colon cancer

*-Having suffered from breast cancer

*-Having polyps in the colon

*-Suffering from ulcerative colitis or Crohn's Disease

The main warning signs that may lead one to suspect the existence of colon cancer are the following:

*-Presence of blood in the stool

*-Changes in evacuation habits

*-Constipation with reduced stool thickness

*-Black or very dark excrements

*-Feeling of defecating after having evacuated

*-Persistent fatigue and weakness of unknown cause

*-Colic and/or persistent abdominal pain

*-Unexplained weight loss

Early colon cancer screening should be done starting at age 50 and at least once every two years. It consists of carrying out two tests:

*-Hidden blood in feces

*-Fecal calprotectin

If the presence of blood is demonstrated in the stool and/or the calprotectin is greater than 50 mg, the patient should be taken for a colonoscopy to investigate the cause of these alterations.

Imaging tests used to diagnose and determine the extent of colon cancer include:

*-Colonoscopy: to visualize and biopsy the tumor in the colon

*-Tomography or Scanner: to evaluate if the tumor has spread

*-MRI: to evaluate the local extension of the tumor

*-CT colonography: if it was not possible to perform the colonoscopy.

If you have been diagnosed with colon cancer, your doctor may recommend certain tests to determine the extent (stage) of the cancer. Stage classification helps determine which treatments are most appropriate for you. In many cases, the stage of the cancer may not be fully determined until after colon cancer surgery.

In the lower stages, the cancer is limited to the lining of the inside of the colon. When it reaches stage IV, the cancer is considered advanced and has spread (metastasized) to other areas of the body.

Colon cancer treatment depends on the stage or severity of the tumor. The treatment possibilities are:

1.-Polypectomy: removal of a small malignant polyp during colonoscopy.

2.-Mucosectomy: it is the removal of a large polyp that includes a portion of the colon mucosa, using colonoscopy.

3.-Laparoscopy: it is a minimal abdominal surgery to remove polyps that could not be removed by colonoscopy.

4.-Hemicolectomy: it is the removal of half of the colon (right, transverse or left) when the tumor is advanced. It also includes the removal of lymph nodes suspected of metastasis.

Chemotherapy uses drugs to kill cancer cells, usually given after surgery if the cancer is large or has spread to the lymph nodes. In this way, chemotherapy can kill any cancer cells that remain in the body and help reduce the risk of cancer recurrence. Chemotherapy may also be used before surgery to shrink a large cancer, so it is easier to remove with surgery.

Chemotherapy may also be used to relieve symptoms of colon cancer that cannot be removed with surgery or that has spread to other parts of the body. Sometimes it is combined with radiotherapy.

Radiation therapy uses powerful energy sources, such as x-rays and protons, to destroy cancer cells. It may be used to shrink a large cancer before an operation so it can be removed more easily. When surgery is not an option, radiation therapy may be used to relieve symptoms, such as pain.

Immunotherapy is a drug treatment that uses your immune system to fight cancer. Your body's disease-fighting immune system may not attack the cancer because cancer cells make proteins that prevent immune system cells from recognizing cancer cells. Immunotherapy works by interfering with that process and is generally reserved for advanced colon cancer. Your doctor may order tests to see if your cancer cells are likely to respond to this treatment.

Palliative care is specialized medical care that focuses on providing relief from pain and other symptoms of a serious illness. Palliative care teams aim to improve the quality of life of people with cancer and their families. This form of care is offered along with curative treatments. When palliative care is used along with all other appropriate treatments, people with cancer can feel better and live longer.

What does non-conventional medicine think?

Integrative Oncology combines the knowledge of official oncology with that of traditional and complementary medicines with proven scientific evidence.

The selection of treatments is carried out seeking satisfactory scientific foundations.

There is scientific evidence on the benefits of acupuncture, herbal medicine, and other complementary therapies to alleviate the symptoms of the side effects of chemotherapy and radiotherapy. Thanks to the combination of both types of treatment, chemotherapy cycles are better tolerated without the need to interrupt them due to decreased immunity or serious side effects.

From the vision of Integrative Oncology, we consider the relationship between the tumor cell and the extracellular space to be of special importance. It has been scientifically proven that when we modify the conditions of the extracellular space, the behavior of tumor cells is modified. It is not enough to attack the tumor cell, it is also necessary to nourish, detoxify, oxygenate, and normalize the pH of the extracellular space, so that once the chemotherapy and radiotherapy treatment cycles are finished, the body is in the most optimal state to avoid recurrences. tumors.

From Integrative Oncology, we consider it extremely important to enhance the immune system, because it is essential for the control of tumor growth as has also been scientifically proven.

With chemotherapy treatments, immunity is greatly affected, therefore it is essential to try to recover it as quickly as possible. To achieve this, Integrative Oncology uses phytotherapy, acupuncture, orthomolecular medicine (vitamins, minerals, amino acids, coenzymes, and probiotics), nutrition, among others.

It is also considered essential to normalize blood levels of stress-related hormones, since it has been proven that some tumors have adrenaline receptors in their membranes and by binding to them, the growth of tumor cells and their ability to produce metastasis.

For this reason, in integrative oncology, much importance is given to mind-body techniques such as yoga or meditation and acupuncture to regulate stress. In the US, some hospitals of recognized prestige in oncology already have an Integrative Oncology department, such as Sloan Kettering Cancer Center, and MD Anderson Cancer Center, among others.

What was the treatment received by Philip?

Philip completed 2 cycles of chemotherapy (Folfox) per month, for a period of six months, for a total of 12 cycles, and each cycle lasted three days.

From the point of view of Complementary Therapy, following the approach of Integrative Oncology, Felipe received two types of treatment:

a-Outpatient:

- Anti-cancer diet and nutrition
- Alkaline anti-cancer juice therapy
- Natural anti-cancer supplements
- Anti-cancer psychological support

b.-Admitted to Clinic:

- B complex, minerals and intravenous trace elements
- Intravenous Vitamin C and Glutathione
- Intravenous hydrogen peroxide and DMSO

All complementary treatment was provided throughout the six months that his chemotherapy lasted and was only suspended 48 hours before and after it to avoid interactions.

What was Philip's clinical evolution?

Felipe evolved excellently, judging by the results obtained:

*-He did not present the classic side effects of chemotherapy such as hair loss, nausea, vomiting, diarrhea, abdominal pain, and mouth sores. He only had some loss of sensation in his hands and feet in the last 2 months.

*-He always maintained his blood values (hemoglobin, leukocytes, and platelets) within normal values and for this reason no chemotherapy treatment was ever suspended.

* -The control CT scan performed in August 2018 did not show the presence of tumor, neither in the colon nor in the lymph nodes, and the two metastases he had in the liver had disappeared.

Given these results, the treating oncologists decided to suspend chemotherapy. Then they planned a quarterly follow-up with PECT-CT that was carried out in November 2018 and then in February 2019, observing the same results. Finally, he underwent annual follow-up, with his last PEC-CT scan being in February 2020, which showed clinical stability without suspicion of tumor recurrence or metastasis.

Conclusion and Discussion

Conventional Oncology maintains its staunch position that the cancer patient should not receive any kind of complementary supportive treatment while receiving treatment based on chemotherapy, immunotherapy, or radiotherapy.

In fact, most oncologists tell their patients, and even give it to them in writing, that during their cancer treatment they should not take any vitamins, minerals, antioxidants, medicinal plants, etc., since these treatments can affect the effects of chemotherapy and even strengthen malignant cells and make them more resistant to treatment.

In contrast, a new medical modality called *Integrative Oncology* has been developed, supported by multiple scientific research, publishing of books and magazines, holding of international scientific events, academic training courses and creation of hospital centers in the main cities of many countries in the world.

There are also publications of books written by doctors who have survived cancer after incorporating complementary therapies. Some of these doctors have even become internationally recognized lecturers.

Philip's clinical case reflects the benefits that an oncology patient can receive, who, in addition to his conventional treatment of surgery and chemotherapy, also received complementary treatment, managing to go through the 6 months of chemotherapy without reflecting relevant side effects and achieve eradication of the signs of metastasis seen in his first post-surgery PEC-CT.

The contrast between these two treatment approaches in cancer patients is somewhat scandalous. It is unacceptable that patients must go to a private center to receive this type of complementary treatments, the effectiveness of which has been demonstrated in thousands of scientific publications and medical research centers of international prestige.

Why the Oncology services of conventional hospitals not only do not accept this scientific evidence, which is disseminated in many countries, but also disqualify, block, and even assume a rebellious and radical position against it, regardless of the benefits it brings can contribute to patients in terms of quality of life, saving suffering and lengthening survival.

We only must ask ourselves a series of questions to invite each reader to reflect, and not fall into the realm of speculation:

1.-If there is so much scientific evidence from different countries, hospitals, research doctors and international organizations, which demonstrates the benefits of the integrative approach in oncological treatment: Why is conventional oncology practiced in most public hospitals, which depend on a government budget, and which take in the vast majority of these patients, does not accept this evidence and does not incorporate this treatment approach on a regular basis?

2.-Where is in all this debate, the right of cancer patients to receive a type of treatment that guarantees the minimum possible side effects, allows them to enjoy a good quality of life and improve the survival prognosis of a disease as impactful and devastating as cancer is?

3.-Where is the individual responsibility of each conventional doctor, who, by ethical mandate, is obliged to stay updated on the advances in medicine, to offer their patients, the most effective and beneficial treatments possible, with the aim of guarantee a good quality of life and overcoming the disease, whenever possible.

4.-Why do the Medical Associations not take on the debate raised around this issue, and based on the principles postulated in the Code of Ethics, which doctors must comply with, do they not defend the rights of cancer patients to receive the benefits of a fairer and more humanized medical approach?

5.- Why does the World Health Organization, which has established specific guidelines for the incorporation of complementary therapies in official health systems in the period from 2011 to 2023, not assume a clear and definitive position on the issue of Integrative Oncology?

6.- Why do the political leaders who direct the governments of the democratic countries of the West not enforce the constitutional mandate of the inalienable right to health, and legislate around the issue of the treatment of cancer patients in all public hospitals?

7.-Are there large-scale economic interests hidden behind this debate, since the pharmaceutical companies that manufacture chemotherapeutic drugs see the practice of Integrative Oncology as a serious threat to their multimillion-dollar profits?

Chapter 9

Esteban's ADHD worries us.

Esteban is a young 15-year-old adolescent who had been taking 2 psychotropic medications (*Rubifen and Concerta*) for 3 years that were prescribed to him by the psychiatrist who had diagnosed him with *Attention Deficit Hyperactivity Disorder* (ADHD), based on the following history reported for his parents:

.-They couldn't keep him still in class, he sang and moved a lot.

.-Poor school performance, he reached the age of 8 without knowing how to read.

.- He repeated the sixth (6th) grade of primary school.

.-At home it was always a conflict for him to start studying.

.- He received help from a Psych pedagogue for 4 years.

.- He passed the first year of secondary education with difficulty

.- He is currently in the 2nd year of secondary education with many difficulties in academic performance

The parents brought him to my office because Esteban was experiencing side effects from the medication, he fell asleep everywhere, nothing sparked his interest, he had very little appetite, weight loss, very frequent headaches, tachycardia, and nervousness.

Taking advantage of the fact that every year the doctor suspends his medication for 4 months during the summer vacation period, his parents wanted to try a different treatment for Esteban's disorder, one that would not entail so many side effects that would affect his quality of life, as was happening to him with the psychiatric treatment he was following.

What does Conventional Medicine think?

Attention-deficit/hyperactivity disorder (ADHD) is a chronic condition that affects millions of children and often continues into adulthood. Risk factors for ADHD may include:

*-Blood relatives, parents, or siblings, with ADHD or another mental health disorder

*-Exposure to environmental toxins, such as lead, found primarily in paint and pipes

*-Use of drugs, alcohol or smoking by the mother during pregnancy

*-Premature birth

Although the exact cause of ADHD is unclear, research continues. Factors that may be involved in the development of ADHD include genetics, the environment, or problems with the central nervous system at key times in development.

There are three subtypes of ADHD:

*-Predominant lack of attention, represents 56% of cases

*-Predominant hyperactive/impulsive behavior. 8% of cases

*-Combined. It represents 36% of cases.

ADHD does not cause other psychological or developmental problems. However, children with ADHD are more likely than others to have conditions such as:

• Oppositional defiant disorder, towards authority figures

• Antisocial behavior disorder

• Disruptive mood dysregulation disorder

• Learning, reading, writing, and communication disabilities

*Substance abuse, including drugs, alcohol, and smoking

• Anxiety disorders and obsessive-compulsive disorder (OCD)

• Mood disorders, including depression and bipolar

• Autism spectrum disorder (ASD)

• Nervous tic or Tourette syndrome.

ADHD can make life difficult for children, because:

• Often fight in the classroom, which can lead to academic failure and judgment from other children and adults

• They tend to have more accidents and injuries of all kinds than children who do not have ADHD

• They tend to have low self-esteem

• Are more likely to have problems interacting with and being accepted by peers and adults

• Are at higher risk for alcohol and drug abuse and other criminal behavior

Generally, a child should not receive a diagnosis of ADHD unless the core symptoms begin early in life (before age 12) and create significant problems at home and at school on an ongoing basis.

There is no specific test for ADHD, but the task of diagnosing is likely to include a medical examination, information gathering, interviews or questionnaires, application of the *Diagnostic and Statistical Manual of Mental Disorders* (DSM-5) criteria for ADHD.

Several medical conditions or their treatments can cause signs and symptoms like those of attention-deficit/hyperactivity disorder.

For example:
• Learning or language problems
• Mood disorders, such as depression or anxiety
• Seizure disorders
• Vision or hearing problems
• Autism spectrum disorder
• Medical problems or medications that affect behavior
• Sleep disorders
• Brain injury

Standard treatments for ADHD in children include:
• Medicines,
• Behavioral therapy,
• Advice,
• Educational services.

These treatments can relieve many of the symptoms of ADHD, but they do not cure it. It may take a while to determine what works best for your child.

Currently, psychostimulant medications are the most prescribed to treat ADHD.

- Amphetamines: Dexedrine or Vyvance
- Methylphenidate: Ritalin or Concerta

Some research indicates that the use of ADHD stimulant medications in patients with certain heart problems may be a concern. The risk of certain psychiatric symptoms may increase when using stimulant medications.

What does non-conventional medicine think?

Children with ADHD often benefit from psychotherapy, social skills training, parenting skills training, and counseling, which may be provided by a psychiatrist, psychologist, social worker, or other mental health professional. Some children with ADHD may also have other conditions such as an anxiety disorder or depression. In these cases, counseling can be helpful for both the ADHD and the co-occurring problem. Some types of these therapies include:

- Family therapy
- Behavioral Psychotherapy
- Parental training
- Social training
- Child psychotherapy

Why should parents try behavioral therapy first before trying any medication?

*-Behavioral therapy gives parents the skills and strategies to help their child.

*-Behavioral therapy has been shown to be as effective as medications in treating ADHD in young children.

*-Young children have more side effects from ADHD medications than older children.

*-The long-term effects of ADHD medications in young children have not been well studied.

In 2010, the Agency for Healthcare Research and Quality (AHRQ) reviewed all existing studies on treatment options for preschool-aged children with ADHD.

The review found sufficient evidence to recommend parent training in behavioral therapy as a good treatment option for children under 6 years of age with ADHD symptoms and for disruptive behaviors in general.

The review also identified four programs for parents of young children with ADHD that reduced ADHD-related symptoms and problem behaviors:

- *Triple P* Positive Parenting Program.
- *Incredible Years* parenting program.
- Parent-child interaction therapy.
- Parenting program for parents of children with ADHD.

There are some studies that have reported the relationship between ADHD and certain foods:

1.-The 5 foods that should be avoided in ADHD

- Sugar: produces hyperactivity
- Gluten: intolerance causes ADHD
- Milk: lactose intolerance affects the brain
- Additives: dyes cause hyperactivity
- Artificial sweeteners: increase ADHD risk

2.- The 5 foods that should be included:

- Omega 3: improve behavior and memory
- Iron: reduces hyperactivity
- Probiotics: prevents Neuroinflammation
- Proteins: improves focus and concentration
- B Complex: reduces ADHD symptoms

In recent years, acupuncture has become a popular complementary therapy for children suffering from ADHD. Auricular acupuncture, specifically, has been shown to be more effective. Since the ear can be stimulated through non-invasive procedures, it is the preferred treatment for children. The ear can be used alone or in combination with body acupuncture through the stimulation of specific points with needles, electricity, lasers, or other devices.

Chinese herbology and acupuncture are often the first choice for children with ADHD, due to the safe nature of the therapies. Since 1980 there have been numerous clinical trials using Chinese herbs alone to help children with ADHD, most of those trials reporting encouraging results. Other studies have shown that acupuncture achieves relatively good clinical efficacy in the treatment of ADHD, particularly for hyperactive and mixed subtypes. Furthermore, recurrence rates after treatment are low. Therefore, this is a type of effective treatment for this disorder, which deserves to be popularized.

What was the treatment followed by Esteban?

When I started working with Esteban, the first thing I observed was that his diet contained:

.-Abundant consumption of cow's milk and various dairy derivatives such as cheese, butter, yogurt, etc.

.-Abundant consumption of red meat, sausages, and hamburgers

.-Abundant consumption of sweets loaded with coloring and food additives

.-Abundant consumption of carbonated drinks such as Coca-Cola and similar.

Considering that the medical literature has reported that there is a close relationship between:

a.-The consumption of sugary foods, loaded with artificial sweeteners and certain colorings added as additives, such as tartrazine, cochineal red, aspartame and orthophosphoric acid, and a higher incidence of ADHD, with a lower response to conventional treatment.

b.-The lack of certain specific nutrients such as B vitamins, vitamin D, amino acids such as tryptophan and omega 3 fatty acids, especially DHA, represents a risk factor for suffering from ADHD.

We decided to follow the following treatment:

*-Implement a gluten-free, FODMAP-type diet, eliminating excess fermentative sugars, in addition to replacing dairy products, red meats and sausages with vegetable and organic alternatives.

*- Include a scheme of nutritional supplements seeking to improve your general and brain nutritional status and observe the impact of this measure on the evolution of your ADHD symptoms.

Finally we included a weekly acupuncture session for the first 2 months and then every 15 days for the next 2 months, for a total of 4 months of treatment.

What was Esteban's evolution with this treatment?

After completing the first four months of treatment we observed a series of clinical changes in Esteban.

*-He recovered his appetite and gained 5 kilograms in the four months that the treatment lasted.

*-There were no headache episodes at any time during the duration of treatment.

*-Fatigue, tiredness, and lack of energy that prevented him from doing sports disappeared

*-Less anxiety and nervousness were recorded when carrying out routine daily activities.

*-Significantly improved the sensation of hyperactivity and showed improvement in concentration and memory.

After observing this clinical improvement in Esteban, his parents decided not to return to the psychotropic medication he was previously taking, after he resumed regular school classes. After a year of follow-up with stability in symptoms and improvement in academic performance, he was discharged from the medical clinic.

Conclusions and Discussion

ADHD is a diagnosis that has been increasing rapidly in recent decades. It is perhaps the most common diagnosis given to children in the United States. More than 10% of boys and 5% of girls suffer from this disorder, according to the American Academy of Child and Adolescent Psychology (AACAP).

Currently, some children diagnosed with ADHD were not actually ADHD, they were simply so happy or intelligent children, who exceeded the ability to handle and understand an increasingly intolerant educational system.

A large part of the parents who have a child with this problem have the feeling that the educational system is using this diagnosis to *label* any child who deviates from the norm, is too restless, and represents a greater workload. for teachers, who, it seems, reflect an increasingly lower level of tolerance, and prefer to deal with a classroom of children high on Ritalin, than with one full of normal, healthy, restless, and energetic children, who demand greater attention, dedication and good teaching on the part of their teachers.

It seems that the diagnosis of ADHD is being abused and Psychiatrists are happy to label all children who are referred by the educational system with this disorder so that they can be prescribed a medication that keeps them sitting in their chairs and does not give them too much work to their teachers.

The conventional treatment of ADHD is through the prescription of the stimulant *methylphenidate* (Ritalin), the production of which has increased sevenfold in the 1990s alone and is continually administered to increasingly younger patients.

The element that arouses great concern to the parents of these children who take psychostimulants are their side effects. On the one hand, they can cause physical disorders, such as dry mouth, nausea, insomnia, palpitations, digestive discomfort, fatigue, loss of appetite and skin spots, which affect the child's quality of life.

On the other hand, they can also cause or exacerbate other psychiatric disorders such as depression, suicidal behavior, hostility, psychosis, and mania.

In the long term, many parents find themselves trapped in the trap of drug dependence and in the sad reality that in seeking to help their children and please their teachers, they end up exchanging a mild psychiatric disorder, ADHD, for another much more serious one, such as severe depression or childhood psychosis.

It is highly regrettable that despite the fact that there are many publications, based on serious scientific studies, of the effectiveness of the combined treatment of dietary changes, supportive nutritional supplementation to modulate brain chemical neurotransmission, and therapy to balance the intestinal microbiota and regulate the functions of the so-called gut-brain axis; Most psychiatrists limit themselves to instituting only standard pharmacological treatment, and almost never explore other options, such as complementary treatments and behavioral psychological therapies that have also been of great help in the management of these children.

The final result of Esteban's story is that he became a child again and recovered the splendor of his childhood, which had been taken from him by the combination of an intolerant educational system and an orthodox psychiatrist, who limited himself to indicating psychotropic treatment. , without considering other forms of less aggressive treatments, and the most serious and painful thing is that he never cared about the terrible side effects that filled the life of this child and his family with sadness.

Chapter 10

Yadira has lost a lot of weight.

Yadira is a 36-year-old woman who, in May 2017, was diagnosed with a digestive infection due to helicobacter pylori and prescribed antibiotic treatment (Pylera) for 10 days. A week after completing this treatment, she began to experience itching all over her body, enlarged lymph nodes in her neck, and progressive and generalized muscle and joint pain. After a couple of weeks, digestive discomfort appeared, gas, flatulence, burning sensation in the stomach, intestinal swelling, and a progressive intolerance to an increasing number of foods, which is why the quantity and type of foods were restricted that she ate daily.

She subsequently began to lose weight slowly and at that point she decided to consult the doctor. Between June and December 2017, she was evaluated by a family doctor, an internist, a neurologist and environmental medicine. She underwent a wide variety of laboratory tests, including sophisticated biochemical tests, determination of heavy metals and minerals in the hair roots, microbiota study and genetic analysis for Celiac disease, rheumatological and immunological tests and gastroscopy.

Yadira visited us in March 2018, she was extremely thin, looked pale and malnourished, she only weighed 35 kilos for a height of 1.56cm.

She wore a mask, had fluid retention and some bruising on her lower extremities, complained of pain all over her body and said that she came because she had been diagnosed with *Fibromyalgia, Chronic Fatigue Syndrome and Multiple Chemical Sensitivity Syndrome.*

She had a very restricted diet with few foods and had tried multiple pharmacological and natural treatments and could not tolerate any of them due to his chemical sensitivity. She commented that she could only tolerate the new supplements for a week and after that time he would begin to reject them with a series of symptoms. She also commented that she had researched the three pathologies that had been diagnosed on the Internet and that all the symptoms coincided with those she had and that all the doctors visited had tried different treatments, including the administration of intravenous vitamins and minerals without achieving any improvement.

There were three aspects that caught our attention about her clinical history, which were the following:

a.-We noticed that Yadira spent 2 hours in the consultation, within a medical establishment, where there were patients, doctors, and nurses, with multiple odors and exposure to varied environmental stimuli and had not expressed any discomfort, even without wearing the mask. This made us doubt the diagnosis of "Multiple Chemical Sensitivity".

b.-We found Yadira very well informed about the three diagnoses that she had been given and she practically recited all the symptoms that she had read on the Internet.

c.-We noticed inconsistencies between what the patient pointed out, what her spouse said, and what she said in the medical reports she presented.

This raised doubts in us about the certainty of her diagnosis.

In view of these observations, we decided to do a small experiment. We prepared 3 small containers with water and told the patient that we needed to do a sensitivity test, in order to plan a possible treatment, we presented the three bottles listed, as follows:

- Bottle #1: we told you it contained a Homeopathic remedy
- Bottle #2: we told you it contained multiminerals.

- Bottle #3: we told you it contained B vitamins.

After tasting the contents of each of the bottles, with a difference of 30 minutes between each one, Yadira experienced the following symptoms:
- Bottle # 1: it caused burning of the scalp and burning of the skin
- Bottle #2: it caused pressure in the head and burning in the stomach
- Bottle #3: it caused pressure in the esophagus and generalized chills

At the end of the experiment, Yadira commented that in view of the reactions she had experienced, it was evident that she could not receive treatment with any of the tested contents, and finally she asked: What type of treatment were we planning to solve her serious and complex pathologies, if she couldn't tolerate practically any substance?

Then we revealed to Yadira that the three jars in the experiment only contained water and therefore, there was no physical explanation for the symptoms that she had felt when testing their contents, and that for that reason we were inclined to think that the root of his illnesses was not in his body but in his mind and in view of this, it seemed to us that the first step should be a visit to the psychologist to evaluate the possibility that it was a case of *Anorexia Nervosa*.

What does Conventional Medicine think?

Fibromyalgia is a disorder characterized by widespread musculoskeletal pain accompanied by fatigue, sleep, memory, and mood problems. Researchers believe that fibromyalgia amplifies painful sensations by affecting the way your brain processes pain signals. Symptoms sometimes begin after physical trauma, surgery, infection, or significant psychological stress. In other cases, symptoms gradually build up over time without a single triggering event. Women are more likely to develop fibromyalgia than men.

Many people who have fibromyalgia also have tension headaches, temporomandibular joint (TMJ) disorders, irritable bowel syndrome, anxiety, and depression. While there is no cure for fibromyalgia, a variety of medications can help manage symptoms. Exercise, relaxation, and stress reduction measures can also help.

Chronic Fatigue Syndrome is a complex disorder characterized by extreme fatigue that cannot be attributed to any pre-existing illness. Fatigue may worsen with physical or mental activity, but it does not improve with rest.

This condition is also known as *systemic exercise intolerance disease* or *myalgic encephalomyelitis*. Sometimes it is abbreviated ME/CFS. The cause of chronic fatigue syndrome is unknown, although there are many theories, ranging from viral infections to psychological stress. Some experts believe that chronic fatigue syndrome can be triggered by a combination of factors.

Multiple chemical sensitivity is a chronic syndrome of unknown origin, in which the patient experiences a wide variety of recurrent symptoms, involving several organs and systems, related to exposure to various substances in very low doses, such as foods or products environmental chemicals. Symptoms may improve when exposure to them is avoided. It usually affects middle-aged women and develops in an overlapping and progressive manner. It is also usually accompanied by food, pharmacological and other types of intolerances. It frequently presents with associated diseases, especially chronic fatigue syndrome.

What does non-conventional medicine think?

Anorexia nervosa is an eating disorder characterized by abnormally low body weight, an intense fear of gaining weight, and a distorted perception of weight. People with anorexia place a high value on controlling their weight and shape, making extreme efforts that tend to significantly interfere with their lives. No matter how much weight is lost, the person continues to fear weight gain. Anorexia is not really about food. It is an extremely unhealthy and sometimes life-threatening way of trying to cope with emotional problems. When you have anorexia, you often equate thinness with self-esteem.

The exact cause of anorexia is unknown, it is probably a combination of biological, psychological, and environmental factors.

Biological. There may be genetic changes that make some people at higher risk of developing anorexia. Some people may have a genetic tendency toward perfectionism, sensitivity, and perseverance, all traits associated with anorexia.

Psychological. Some people with anorexia may have obsessive-compulsive personality traits that make it easy to follow strict diets and give up food despite being hungry. They may have an extreme drive for perfectionism, causing them to think that they are never thin enough. And they may have high levels of anxiety and engage in restrictive eating to reduce it.

Environmental. Modern Western culture emphasizes thinness. Success and worth are often equated with being thin. Peer pressure can help fuel the desire to be thin, especially among girls.

Physical signs and symptoms of anorexia may include:
- Extreme weight loss
- Slim appearance
- Abnormal blood counts
- Fatigue, insomnia, dizziness, or fainting
- Bluish discoloration of the fingers.
- Hair that thins, breaks, or falls out
- Soft, downy hair that covers the body.
- Absence of menstruation
- Constipation and abdominal pain.
- Dry or yellowish skin
- Cold intolerance
- Irregular heart rhythms

- Low blood pressure
- Dehydration
- Swelling of arms or legs

Emotional and behavioral signs and symptoms may include:

- Concern about food,
- Skipping meals frequently or refusing to eat
- Denial of hunger or excuses for not eating
- Eat only some "safe" foods
- Adopt rigid meals or eating rituals
- Not wanting to eat in public
- Lying about how much food has been eaten
- Fear of gaining weight and weigh themselves repeatedly
- Frequent checking in the mirror for defects
- Complaining about being fat or having fat body parts
- Cover yourself with layers of clothing
- Flat mood (lack of emotion)
- Social withdrawal, irritability, and insomnia
- Reduced interest in sex

Anorexia can have numerous complications, such as:

- Anemia
- Mitral valve prolapse, arrhythmias or heart failure
- Bone loss (osteoporosis), which increases the risk of fractures.
- Muscle loss
- In women, absence of period
- In men, decreased testosterone.
- Gastrointestinal, such as constipation, bloating, or nausea.
- Low potassium, sodium, and chloride in the blood
- Kidney problems

People with anorexia also often have other mental health disorders. They may include:

- Depression, anxiety, and other mood disorders.
- Obsessive compulsive disorders

- Alcohol and substance abuse
- Self-harm, suicidal thoughts, or suicide attempts.

Treatment for anorexia is typically done through a team approach, including doctors, mental health professionals, and dietitians, all with experience in eating disorders. Ongoing therapy and nutritional education are very important for continued recovery.

The first goal of treatment is to regain a healthy weight. You cannot recover from anorexia without returning to a healthy weight and learning proper nutrition. Those involved in this process may include:

* -His family, who will likely be involved in helping him maintain normal eating habits

*- Your primary care doctor, to provide you with medical care and monitor your caloric needs and weight gain.

*- A dietician, who can offer guidance on returning to regular eating patterns, including providing specific meal plans and caloric requirements to help you achieve your weight goals.

*- A psychologist or other mental health professional who can work with you to develop behavioral strategies to help you regain a healthy weight.

One of the biggest challenges in treating anorexia is that people may not want treatment. Barriers to treatment may include:

- Thinking you don't need treatment
- Fearing weight gain
- Do not see anorexia as a disease, but as a lifestyle choice.

People with anorexia can recover. However, they are at higher risk of relapse during periods of high stress or during triggering situations. Ongoing therapy or regular appointments during times of stress can help you stay healthy.

What was Yadira's treatment and evolution?

Yadira was evaluated by the health team's psychologist who, after five sessions, issued the following report:

.-Yadira comes from a home with too much overprotection and has a 3-year-old daughter with whom she repeats the same scheme of overprotection.

.- Since she was a child she learned to hide her feelings, she developed many fears, insecurity, doubts, etc., and took control through weight and food.

.-She tends to have unrealistic expectations of herself and other people around her such as parents, siblings and friends.

.- Despite being successful in her job and family, she feels incapable of running the home, inept, defective, and has no sense of identity, and that is why she tries to take control of her life by focusing on her physical appearance to obtain that control.

.- She experiences marked social isolation, excessive tiredness, sleepiness, irritability, aggression (especially towards the mother figure), shame, guilt and depression.

.-The patient has developed an *Eating Disorder* (ED), basing all her thoughts and actions that are part of her daily life on food, feeling hyper dependent on that idea, with which food has become the axis from which your life and your world of relationships revolve.

.-The final conclusion is that it is a picture of *Anorexia Nervosa* where the excessive and obsessive concern about one's physical figure and weight have been masked by the supposed *Fibromialgia, Chronic Fatigue Syndrome* and *Multiple Chemical Sensitivity Syndrome* that she was diagnosed with.

Based on the psychologist's conclusion, we designed an integrative treatment approach based on:

a.-Psychological Treatment; aimed at achieving lasting changes in distorted thoughts and negative emotions related to weight, shape, and body size in their value system to build or recover an identity that helps the patient feel good about themselves, so as not to have to resort to food control/lack of control in the face of the challenges and problems that life poses.

.-The patient's self-esteem was promoted in each session

.-She was helped to find his own values, ideals and objectives without being influenced by the environment

.-The family was guided to communicate to the patient, clearly, the concern felt for her, the conviction that she needs treatment, and the willingness to provide her with emotional, financial or any other type of support.

.-Avoid concentrating on her appearance. Comments like "you're too thin!" or "come on, you're really skinny!" They can only make the patient more obsessed with her bodily appearance.

.-Do not force her to eat, nor criticize her attitudes, as that will probably increase her depression and make her obsess over her behavior. You need to be patient.

.- Do not establish comparisons between the patient and the people around her

-Try to ensure that the situation does not alter family life. Do not leave aside your own family.

.-Avoid feelings of guilt or self-pity.

.- We worked on re-educating the patient in judicious eating habits, maintaining a relaxed and natural person-food relationship.

.-We worked to avoid self-destructive thoughts and unrealistic points of view about the food-appearance-happiness relationship.

b.-Nutritional Treatment; A balanced and healthy diet was planned, with a 4-week rotating menu to avoid food intolerance. In addition, nutritional supplementation was provided to recover the nutritional deficiencies that were detected in the tests, such as hypovitaminosis D, B12, anemia, etc.

c.-Medical Treatment; Monthly medical follow-up was implemented to monitor clinical and laboratory evolution, ensuring nutritional recovery, weight gain and stabilization of all organic functions, avoiding damage to any organ due to nutrient deficiency.

The patient's evolution was highly satisfactory and her nutritional and psychological recovery was progressive over the course of the eight months that her treatment lasted, reaching her ideal weight, the recovery of all observed nutritional deficiencies and the normalization of all laboratory variables. The patient was evaluated quarterly in 2019 and in view of there being no relapses and remaining normal, she was discharged in January 2020.

Conclusions and Discussion

a.-In 1970 the World Health Organization (WHO) defined Health as: *"The complete state of biological, psychological and social well-being, and not only the absence of disease."* However, conventional medicine maintains its biological approach and almost never considers psychological and social aspects in the etiology and treatment of the disease.

b.-This clinical case dramatically illustrates this reality. Yadira spent nine months rotating from doctor to doctor, undergoing endless expensive laboratory tests and undergoing various types of treatments without obtaining favorable results, because the root of her problem was in her mind and not in her body, and none of the Doctors consulted in those nine months considered that possibility.

c.-The integrative therapeutic approach where the psychological, nutritional, and medical aspects were managed simultaneously and progressively managed to recover Yadira from her health disorder and insert her into her normal life after eight months of treatment.

d.-It is also important to highlight that Yadira never suffered from Fibromyalgia, Chronic Fatigue Syndrome and Multiple Chemical Sensitivity Syndrome.

They were only labels placed by the doctors consulted, who were unable to distinguish that most of the symptoms reported by Yadira were part of her eating disorder and not specific medical pathologies such as those indicated, which, far from helping to solve her problem, contributed to increasing it.

e.- Our mind is powerful and the way we manage our emotions directly influences our overall health. Hence the idea that many diseases depend on the interaction between our spirit and our emotions.

These are the so-called psychosomatic diseases. They are defined as those that are caused by stress, tension, radical changes in lifestyle and emotions. There is no doubt that all these factors can influence our physical appearance and cause health problems. Many studies show that our emotions have a decisive influence on heart and mental illnesses, stomach pains, etc. The accumulation of tension often has repercussions on the body.

f.-The best way to control and avoid psychosomatic diseases is to prevent stress and adapt our physical responses to situations that make us nervous or that generate tension.

Observe your emotions and your feelings, the way your body reacts to a crisis or a specific situation. This makes it easier to determine if what we do directly affects our health.

It is essential to carry out activities to combat stress, such as having a hobby or exercising. These are good ways to disconnect and get rid of what causes tension and generates discomfort.

It is very important to learn to resolve conflicts using the emotional intelligence of the affected parties. Psychosomatic illnesses appear very often because we accumulate tensions generated by our problems instead of looking for solutions. It is important to find alternatives to free our spirit and our body from the stress caused by daily problems.

Chapter 11

Luis can no longer cope his Asthma.

Luis is a 36-year-old man, a gardener by trade, who visited me in April 2012 stating that for 2 years he had been suffering from a repetitive pattern of wet cough with yellowish-green expectoration and sometimes with streaks of blood, nasal congestion, and itchy throat, tightness in the chest and feeling of shortness of breath, especially in the mornings. He has been evaluated by a pulmonologist who diagnosed him with recurrent and persistent *chronic rhinopharyngitis and asthmatic bronchitis*, and indicated aerosol-based treatment, vaccine therapy, antiallergy medications, and antibiotics, all of which he has rigorously complied with for more than a year without observing no change in his symptoms. Luis decided to consult me for a second opinion, hoping to find a different solution that would provide him with better results than those obtained so far.

When we took his medical history, Luis gave us the following information:

*-He had no history of allergies in his childhood or adolescence

*-There was no family history of respiratory allergies and asthma

*- There was no history of smoking or other drugs

*-He suffers from 3 episodes of sinusitis a year since he has been a gardener

*-He consumed a lot of dairy products, sausages, fast food, sweets, bottled juices, cookies, and ice cream.

We suspect that there must be an occupational factor that was related to his respiratory symptoms, since he did not have a clear history of familial allergic asthma. For this reason, we performed a series of examinations on Luis, and isolated a fungus from his respiratory tract, called *Aspergillus Nigger.*

With these results we concluded that Luis's respiratory condition corresponded to *Pulmonary Aspergillosis* with involvement of the paranasal sinuses (chronic sinusitis), bronchial sinuses (recurrent bronchitis) and persistent bronchospasm (asthmatiform condition).

What does Conventional Medicine think?

Aspergillosis is an infection caused by a type of mold (fungus). Diseases resulting from aspergillosis infection generally affect the respiratory system, but the signs and severity vary greatly. Aspergillus mold, which triggers illness, is everywhere, both indoors and outdoors. Most strains of this mold are harmless, but a few can cause serious illness when people with weakened immune systems, underlying lung disease, or asthma inhale their fungal spores.

The risk of developing aspergillosis depends on your general health and the degree of exposure to mold. In some people, the spores trigger an allergic reaction. And other people get mild or severe lung infections. The most serious type of aspergillosis occurs when the infection spreads to the blood vessels and beyond. Depending on the type of aspergillosis, treatment may involve observation, antifungal medications, or, in unusual cases, surgery.

People who are exposed to Aspergillus can manifest different clinical symptoms, the most frequent being the following:

1.-Allergic reactions

Some people who have asthma have an allergic reaction to aspergillus mold. Signs and symptoms of this condition, known as *allergic bronchopulmonary aspergillosis*, include:

- Fever
- Cough that may cough up blood or plugs of mucus
- Worsening of asthma

2.-Aspergilloma

It occurs when Aspergillus invades the lung cavities of a person who suffers from emphysema, sarcoidosis, or tuberculosis, forming fungal lumps called *Aspergilloma*, which can cause the following symptoms:

- A cough that can sometimes cough up blood (hemoptysis)
- Wheezing
- Shortness of breath
- Involuntary weight loss
- Fatigue

3.-Invasive Aspergillosis

This is the most serious type of aspergillosis. It occurs when the infection spreads rapidly from the lungs to the brain, heart, kidneys, or skin. *Invasive aspergillosis* only occurs in people whose immune system is weakened because of cancer chemotherapy, bone marrow transplant, or an immune system disease. If left untreated, this type of aspergillosis can be fatal.

The symptoms are:

- Fever, chills, and shortness of breath.
- A cough that produces blood (hemoptysis)
- Chest or joint pain
- Headaches or eye symptoms
- Skin lesions.

The diagnosis of *Aspergillosis* requires several tests, such as chest x-ray, culture of sputum or respiratory secretion, and sometimes even tissue biopsy.

The treatment of *Aspergillosis* requires the use of antifungals to eliminate the fungus and corticosteroids to control the asthmatic allergic reaction. Sometimes surgery may be required to remove Aspergillomas.

What does non-conventional medicine think?

*-Food and respiratory allergies

It happens, without knowing it, that many people with asthma and respiratory allergies suffer serious attacks exacerbated by the consumption of milk and dairy derivatives. Many times, these dairy intolerances cause side effects in which the cause is not identified. The consumption of milk causes in some people intolerant to this food:

fluid retention, difficult digestion, and an increase in the density of mucus that causes respiratory problems.

It may also happen that the intolerance is towards another food that is part of the usual diet and that is causing respiratory crises.

A person with an allergy should not consume foods with more than 20 milligrams per kilo of histamines. Raw milk can have 360 mg, pasteurized milk from 10 to 165 mg and cured cheeses between 500 and 700 mg. Histamine is a highly allergic molecule.

In addition to milk, it is advisable to limit red meat, sausages, smoked, fermented meats, saturated fats, hydrogenated fats, artificial sweeteners, carbonated drinks and preserves in general from the diet.

Make a personalized and balanced diet. Eat a variety of foods, plenty of salads, green leafy vegetables and fruits, white and blue fish, white meats, legumes, and cereals. Vegan food is also another very good option, although fermented soy derivatives have very high levels of histamine.

*-Natural antifungals

Caprylic acid is a type of beneficial saturated fatty acid that has antibacterial, antiviral, antifungal, and anti-inflammatory properties. Along with capric acid and lauric acid, caprylic acid is one of the three primary fatty acids found in coconut oil. Taken internally, it helps naturally reduce the growth of yeast within the gastrointestinal tract while helping beneficial bacteria thrive.

Because caprylic acid acts as a natural fungal fighting agent, it is believed that it can penetrate the cell membranes of cells and cause them to die, detoxifying the digestive tract and speeding up the healing process.

What type of treatment did Luis receive?

Due to the presence of Aspergillus in Luis's sputum samples, we indicated the following treatment:

a.-Nutritional Education

*-Replacement of cow's milk with vegetable drinks based on oats, almonds, and rice

*-Replacement of dairy products with tofu, soy yogurt, and butter

*-Replacement of meat sausages with vegetable derivatives

*-Replacement of coffee with malted cereals based on rooibos

*-Elimination of all types of foods based on fungi and yeasts

*-Fodmap diet to eliminate excess fermentative sugars

b.-Nutritional Supplementation

*-Natural anti-fungal: caprylic acid and wood of arc

*-Natural antibiotics: garlic, grapefruit, and tea tree capsules

*-Bronchial Plants: Eucalyptus, Drossera, Mullein, Boswellia

*-Antioxidants: vitamin C, Selenium, Zinc, lipoic acid

*-Extra virgin vegetable oils: perita oil

c.-Specific anti-fungal medication:

• Itraconazole; 100mg morning and night for 30 days

What was Luis' evolution?

After completing 15 days of pharmacological treatment and two months of nutrition and supplementation, Luis showed excellent medical progress.

The respiratory difficulty disappeared and with it the need to use bronchodilator aerosols, the cough with thick mucus expectoration and the symptoms of sinusitis also improved significantly.

His physical examination showed the disappearance of the bronchial sounds that were noted in the first consultation. Nasal exudate and sputum cultures were negative for fungi and bacteria. Likewise, the control x-ray showed improvement in chronic sinusitis and bronchitis.

Luis was given recommendations to use strict respiratory protection in his work environment to avoid reinfection by fungi and we subjected him to a quarterly medical check-up with X-ray and cultures of nasal exudate and sputum for six months without evidence of any reactivation of the infection. We also recommend maintaining dietary changes and intermittently taking medicinal plants and nutritional supplements,

After 9 months of follow-up, showing stability of the clinical improvement achieved, in addition to verifying Luis's compliance with everything recommended, we discharged him from the clinic.

Conclusions and Discussion

In many hospitals in Europe, and in the world, the doctors who work there are obliged to follow a protocol that has been established by a committee of expert doctors. According to this work model, once the doctor has collected the main symptoms and signs that the patient is experiencing, he must follow what is established by the protocol.

Which in most cases is computerized and to which all doctors who have access, they are part of the staff of each hospital.

The protocol establishes the possible diagnoses for the symptoms and signs noted, indicates the laboratory tests and/or special tests that should be ordered, the medications recommended for that case almost always based on symptomatic relief, and establishes the criteria that the patient must meet to be referred to a specialist or to the medical emergency room, if the case requires it.

All doctors must faithfully follow the protocol every time they treat a patient and when they do not, they must offer a solid and convincing argument, otherwise they will be reprimanded by hospital managers.

The hospital work style based on following the protocol is justified by those who defend it, arguing a series of administrative advantages that it offers, such as:

a.-It helps the doctor to refer each patient quickly, which optimizes the time dedicated to each patient in consultation, and this has made it possible to establish a minimum time per consultation that is between 5 and 10 minutes.

b.-As the protocol system allows optimizing the time that each doctor dedicates to patients, it increases hospital performance in terms of quantity, which is one of the parameters with which hospitals compete to move in a national and international ranking. hospital quality.

c.-The medical system based on the protocol also allows for the optimization of material resources, since doctors must follow the recommendations on laboratory examinations, special tests and indicated medications, avoiding digression and tests requested erratically, especially by the of the youngest doctors.

d.-As the protocol clearly establishes the criteria that the patient must meet to be referred to a specialized consultation or medical emergencies, in theory, it would generate decongestion in both sectors, thus allowing the optimized use of both the contracted time of the specialist doctors , such as the human resources available to the medical emergency room, which operates 24 hours a day, 7 days a week.

e.-Finally, the defenders of the medical model of the protocol affirm that this system allows reducing medical error since there is a unification of criteria, established by the most experienced doctors, and that must be followed by all doctors, especially the youngest and less experienced.

Reality, however, has shown that the protocol-based medical system is far from being an ideal model for the management of hospital patients, and in practice, several drawbacks have arisen that seriously compromise the quality of this system. model of medical care, consequently generating a regrettable deterioration in the nature of the medical care offered and thus compromising the health of patients, often subjecting them to situations that endanger their lives. For example:

a.-As a consequence of having a time allocated per patient, which is around 10 minutes, most doctors have stopped taking a complete medical history, skipping the patient's physical examination.

This type of medical care represents a devirtualization of the medical act itself, which can be very beneficial for the administrative and political purposes of the hospital, but which is totally incoherent and harmful for both the patient and the doctor.

b.-The doctor-patient relationship has been lost, the doctor, therefore, can never get to know his patient well and in this way, the probabilities of falling into medical error are very great.

c.-The medical act has been dehumanized, since what should be a conversation between two people, based on attentive listening and directed interrogation, to obtain precise information, has become the act of filling out a form to follow a guide of steps issued by a computer.

d.-The patient has been stripped of his status as a sick person and has been robbed of his right to be able to speak and explain what he feels, all his symptoms, his fears and anxieties, what he thinks and has deduced from his own discomfort; and instead, he has been converted into an issuer of specific data that is required to provide information to a computer, who, ultimately, will be the one who will dictate the steps to follow, previously established in a precise protocol.

e.-The doctor has been stripped of his status as a health professional, since his ability to think, analyze, contrast, deduce and conclude, based on his theoretical knowledge and his clinical experience, has been denied; and instead, he has been converted into a qualified secretary, whose job is to quickly obtain the main data issued by the patient to fill out a form and obtain a response from a computer indicating the steps to be followed, without right to disagree and much less to deviate from the protocol.

f.-The assertiveness and effectiveness of the medical assistance offered under the protocol model is very poor and mediocre, since by eliminating the true medical act, the conditions are created to fall into medical error or iatrogenesis.

In this way the patients receive treatments that are inappropriate most of the time, and their illnesses reach a critical level, which forces them to seek care in emergency rooms to be hospitalized and resolve by this means what could have been resolved in a medical consultation carried out under the paradigm of a true doctor-patient relationship.

g.-The risk of failing in the objective of solving the problem of the majority of patients, not only generates repeated consultations, in the desperate search for a coherent and assertive response to resolve an illness, with the consequent increase in resource expenditure economic and human; but also, and this is the most serious, it endangers the health and lives of many patients who wander like wandering Jews from consultation to consultation, looking for a solution, while their illnesses advance inexorably, under the pernicious gaze of a system cold, dehumanized and mediocre doctor, leading to complications, seriousness and sometimes death.

Luis's clinical case is a good example of the ineffectiveness of medical care based on protocol. Below we point out the arguments that support this statement:

a.-Luis consulted for respiratory symptoms suggestive of bronchitis and asthma. His family doctor followed the protocol and recommended the indicated treatment based on expectorants, antibiotics, and bronchodilators. Since the patient was not improving, after trying 3 different types of medications, the doctor once again followed the protocol and referred the patient to a specialist.

b.-The Pulmonologist verified that the family doctor followed the protocol, since he referred the patient to his office after trying three different types of treatments.

In turn, the Pulmonologist also followed the protocol, which indicated that the patient's symptoms were highly indicative of chronic sinusitis, acute intermittent bronchitis, bronchial asthma, and added anti-allergy, inhaled corticosteroids, and vaccine therapy to the treatment for several months.

c.-After a year of follow-up, first 3 consultations with the primary care doctor and then another 3 consultations with the Pulmonologist, both doctors following the instructions of the protocol, Luis had not only not improved in his clinical condition, but he was forced to go to the medical emergency room on two occasions due to a worsening of his clinical condition, requiring 48 hours of observation and intravenous medication to stabilize him.

d.-During all that time none of the doctors realized that due to his type of work as a gardener, Luis could have developed an occupational disease, and due to exposure to pollen and dust from different plants, he could have developed a respiratory infection. unusual, which does not respond to common treatments.

e.-As the protocol is rigid and is designed to treat diseases and not people, it does not allow doctors to think about other possibilities and adapt to the individual conditions and characteristics of each patient.

In the case of Luis, it was enough to perform a microbiological study of his secretions, both nasal and pulmonary, to discover the primary cause responsible for all his symptoms, which turned out to be an infection by a fungus (*Aspergillus Nigger*), and to establish a treatment integrative, based on education, medications, supplements and plants, the patient's complete cure was achieved.

The hygienic and preventive measures taught to Luis to put into practice in his work environment and the job rotation recommended to his employer, were effective in keeping him free of reinfection by that fungus and other infectious agents that could affect his respiratory tract. .

Hippocrates, the father of medicine, said in ancient Greece: "*There are no diseases, only the sick, and it is the duty of the doctor to preserve health whenever possible, using all available resources to achieve that goal, always taking care of the maximum, first do no harm.*" Considering the arguments presented, Hippocratic thought, and mandate are incompatible with medical care based on the *protocol.*

Chapter 12

Silvia so young and with Rheumatism

In July 2015, Silvia, a 12-year-old teenager, who enjoyed apparent good health, began to have pain and inflammation in her wrist and some fingers on both hands. She had swelling, stiffness, and great difficulty moving and using her hands. The entire picture was established within a period of 3 weeks. In August she was evaluated by the Rheumatologist, who, after performing some blood tests and an ultrasound of both hands, made the diagnosis of severe *Juvenile Rheumatoid Arthritis* and indicated treatment with Methotrexate, a very powerful medication that usually causes many side effects. To calm the pain, he also recommended conventional anti-inflammatories.

After a year of treatment and quarterly control by Rheumatology, Silvia continued with the same symptoms and already had a discrete deformity of some fingers on her hands. Her response to the treatment had been very poor and for that reason her doctor decided to transfer her to a more aggressive treatment based on *Monoclonal Antibodies*, a therapy that is applied intravenously once a month in the hospital and produces a drastic and persistent suppression of the immune system, seeking to regulate the autoimmunity defect that causes the disease.

Silvia's mother was very concerned about her daughter's illness and before continuing with the new treatment proposed by the rheumatologist, she decided to seek a second opinion.

In the hope of finding a different and less aggressive and risky solution for her daughter.

What does Conventional Medicine think?

Juvenile rheumatoid arthritis, the most common type of arthritis in children under 16 years of age, can cause persistent joint pain, inflammation, and stiffness. Some children may experience symptoms for only a few months, while others have symptoms for the rest of their lives. Some types of juvenile rheumatoid arthritis can cause serious complications, such as growth problems, joint damage, and eye inflammation. Treatment focuses on controlling pain and inflammation, improving function, and preventing joint damage.

Juvenile rheumatoid arthritis can affect one or more joints. There are different subtypes, but the main ones are systemic, which affects the joints and can affect other organs of the body, polyarticular, which affects several joints without affecting other organs, and oligoarticular, which affects only a few joints. Like other forms of arthritis, it is characterized by periods in which symptoms are exacerbated and periods in which they are relieved.

Juvenile rheumatoid arthritis occurs when the body's immune system attacks its own cells and tissues. The reason why this happens is unknown, but both heredity and environment seem to play a role. Some genetic mutations could make a person more sensitive to environmental factors, such as viruses, that could trigger the disease.

The diagnosis of juvenile idiopathic arthritis may be difficult to make since joint pain may be caused by many different types of problems. There is no single test that can confirm the diagnosis, but there are tests that can help rule out other conditions that produce similar signs and symptoms.

Some of the most frequent blood tests in suspected cases include the following:

*-Sedimentation rate, measures the degree of body inflammation

*-C-reactive protein, also measures the level of general inflammation

*-Antinuclear antibodies, measures the patient's autoantibodies

*-Rheumatoid factor, which increases when there is arthritis

*-Anti-cyclic citrullinated peptide antibodies are also elevated.

X-rays or MRI scans are helpful in ruling out other disorders, such as fractures, tumors, infections, and birth defects. Imaging tests are also sometimes used after diagnosis to monitor bone development and detect joint damage.

Treatment of juvenile rheumatoid arthritis focuses on helping the patient maintain a normal level of physical and social activity. To achieve this, doctors could combine strategies to relieve pain and inflammation, maintain full motion and strength, and prevent complications.

Medications used to help children with arthritis are selected to decrease pain, improve function, and minimize potential joint damage. Some of the ones that are usually used are:

*-Nonsteroidal anti-inflammatory drugs (NSAIDs). These medications (aspirin, ibuprofen, etc.) relieve pain and reduce inflammation. Side effects include stomach pain and liver problems.

*-Disease-modifying antirheumatic drugs. Doctors use these drugs when NSAIDs alone fail to relieve disease symptoms or when there is a high risk of future harm. The most used is *Methotrexate* and its side effects could include liver or kidney problems.

*-Corticosteroids. The most common, Prednisone can be used to control symptoms when other medications have had no effect, or when other organs are affected. They can interfere with normal growth and increase susceptibility to infections, so in general they should be used for the shortest time possible.

*-Biological agents. It is a new class of medications that can help reduce systemic inflammation and prevent joint damage. It includes tumor necrosis factor blocking agents, such as Enbrel and Humira, and those that strongly inhibit the immune system, such as Orencia, Rituxan, Kineret and Actemra. Its side effects are very varied and delicate.

The doctor may recommend physical therapy to help keep the joints flexible and maintain range of motion and muscle tone, and an occupational therapist may offer recommendations regarding the best exercise and protective equipment for the patient. He or she may also recommend the use of joint supports or splints to help protect your joints and keep them in a good functional position. Finally, in very severe cases, surgery may be needed to improve the position of a joint.

What does non-conventional medicine think?

Some studies published in recent decades point to a relationship between arthritis, the intestines and diet. *Dr. José Scher*, director of the New York University Arthritis Clinic, discussed four different types of arthritis that are connected to inflammatory responses in the gut, including one related to celiac disease or gluten intolerance. He said he had also seen some of his patients with autoimmune arthritis improve by eliminating gluten from their diet, saying, *"A small 2006 study published in the journal Gut found significantly elevated antibodies to various foods in the digestive tract of patients with rheumatoid arthritis".*

Dr. Julie Segre, principal investigator at the US National Human Genome Research Institute, points out the importance of maintaining a healthy intestine to improve the symptoms of arthritis. In the specific case of the child, eating foods that can inflame the intestine, such as milk and gluten, worsened the symptoms of arthritis; eliminating them made the child improve. Also, the Microbiota is very important to maintain balance in the intestine. For this reason, the use of antibiotics is not recommended, since it eliminates the good bacteria that maintain harmony by not allowing the reproduction of bad bacteria. Some researchers are optimistic that probiotics, which contain various strains of bacteria, could help restore an imbalanced intestinal population. Another potential method of recolonizing the intestine, which is gaining ground, is fecal transplantation.

Gluten is a protein found in most grains. Bread, pasta, and cookies are some of the foods that contain gluten.

Some people who are intolerant to gluten may experience digestive symptoms due to its consumption, but others do not present these symptoms and may therefore excessively increase their consumption and therefore the risk of suffering from rheumatoid arthritis.

Having a gluten intolerance means that the body has difficulty digesting this protein found in grains, such as oats, wheat, barley, rye, and others. If it is not detected in time or managed correctly, we can suffer serious consequences such as diabetes and intestinal cancer. A gluten intolerance can cause joint pain which is also a symptom of rheumatoid arthritis. Other symptoms may include muscle cramps, hair loss, nausea, abdominal pain, loss of appetite, mouth ulcers, and seizures.

Rheumatoid arthritis can be caused by leaky gut syndrome. It consists of certain foods, mainly gluten and milk, causing inflammation in the intestine. This leads to the tight junctions between the cells that make up the intestinal lining becoming loose. Then, the barrier begins to let in undesirable substances, different proteins or bacteria and their metabolites, which begin to leak into the surrounding tissues. Uninvited guests trigger an offensive through the body, which uses inflammation to try to get rid of them. This sustained inflammatory response characterizes autoimmune disease.

Multiple studies have shown that eliminating animal products from your diet improves arthritis symptoms, says *Dr. Heidi Turner* of the Arthritis Clinic in Seattle. *"Because it's plant-based, it's naturally anti-inflammatory,"* she adds. A proper diet can reduce the symptoms of rheumatoid arthritis.

Eliminating foods that trigger an autoimmune response, such as meat, eggs, wheat, oranges, milk, peanuts, malt, and soy, among others, prevents and even delays the progression of the disease.

Studies with rheumatoid arthritis patients show that vegan diets appear to decrease morning stiffness and pain and reduce the release of anti-inflammatory substances that cause joint destruction.

According to nutrition specialist *Dana Pitman*, from the Hospital for Specialized Surgery, in New York:

-"Most people begin to notice improvements about two weeks after starting an anti-inflammatory diet."

-"How significant the change is and how soon you detect it, depends largely on what your diet consists of"

-"If you were full of processed foods and sugar and suddenly switch to a regimen of natural, minimally processed foods, you will feel very bad the first few days because you will be in a period of withdrawal."

-"But once you get over it, you'll feel great. You will have a high level of energy, many people become deflated and feel lighter. "In general, most report higher performance when they get the nutrients the body needs to perform its daily functions."

How did we treat Silvia?

Based on the results of multiple published medical studies that relate the genesis of autoimmune diseases to food intolerances, especially to gluten, and the favorable evolution of Rheumatoid Arthritis with an anti-inflammatory diet free of dairy, meat, and other products of animal origin, we decided to follow these guidelines to treat Silvia.

We thus indicate a treatment based on:

a.-100% gluten-free and FODMAP-type diet free of simple sugars such as lactose, fructose, and sorbitol

b.-Nutritional education, focused on the correct combination of foods, following an order in eating, respecting the 80:20 rule that recommends:

- 80% raw and only 20% cooked
- 80% alkaline and only 20% acids
- 80% whole grain and only 20% refined foods
- 80% fermentative and only 20% putrefactive

c.-Anti-inflammatory medicinal plants, such as devil's claw, turmeric and Boswellia Serratia.

d.-Chondroprotectors based on Glucosamine, Chondroitin, MSM, hyaluronic acid and type II collagen.

e.-Immunomodulators based on Noni juice, Shark Cartilage and Transfer Factors.

We request laboratory tests to investigate:

- Intolerance to gluten, lactose, sorbitol, fructose, and histamine
- Genetic study and IgA antibodies for Celiac disease
- Monitoring of blood erythrocyte sedimentation rates and ANA titers

What was the evolution that Silvia had?

Silvia was followed from November 2016 to January 2019 and her clinical and laboratory evolution was as follows:

a.-The laboratory analyzes carried out reported:

- Negative celiac disease test, ruling out the disease.
- Intolerance to gluten, sorbitol, lactose, and fructose was demonstrated.

b.-The values of the autoantibodies (ANA) and inflammation (ESR) will normalize after 5 months of treatment, with an ANA value of 1/80 and an ESR value of 8mm/hour.

c.-Silvia lost 12 kilos in the first 6 months of treatment and maintained it until she was discharged from the clinic.

d.-The clinical symptoms completely disappeared in 4 months, with complete improvement of the pain and inflammation of the joints of the wrists and fingers. A 100% recovery of hand functionality was recorded.

These clinical results were maintained for two years and until discharge from the clinic in January 2019.

e.-The Ultrasound of the fingers performed in October 2018, two years after starting the integrative treatment, reported discrete thickening of soft tissues in relation to his arthritis. No free fluid is seen around the tendons.

In view of these results, her rheumatologist decided to suspend the methotrexate treatment and only recommended the use of regular analgesics and anti-inflammatory drugs (NSAIDs) as needed and if she needed them. Regarding rheumatology consultations, they were spaced every six months in the first year, and once a year starting in 2018.

Conclusion and Discussion

The medical and nutritional publications that point out the relationship between rheumatoid arthritis and pro-inflammatory diets and with intestinal permeability, intestinal dysbiosis and food intolerances are abundant and overwhelming. Also, for more than a decade, the beneficial impact of vegetarian diets on the course of inflammatory symptoms and the frequency of rheumatoid arthritis attacks has been known. However, in conventional medical practice, in Rheumatology services, both public and private, where the immense population of patients affected by Rheumatoid Arthritis is treated, this universal, scientific, and medically accepted knowledge is not applied in all university centers and prestigious medical associations.

In conventional medical practice, the patient is almost never asked about the foods he regularly eats in his daily life, since this parameter is not included in the formats where the information is collected to prepare the patient's clinical history, and on the other hand, the doctor does not show any interest in knowing about this information because he considers it *irrelevant* to construct his analysis and design his strategic diagnosis and treatment plan.

In the best of cases, if the doctor considers that the diet factor could have some importance in the treatment of a specific pathology, he would make a referral of the patient to a *Nutrition and Dietetics* service, so that the nutrition professional is the one who be in charge of covering that aspect, because the nutritional factor of a patient is definitely not a field in which the doctor can move.

This reality is due, in large part, to the fact that the doctor does not receive any training in nutrition while studying medicine at the university, since most professors, if not all, consider that the medical student must focus on learning to diagnose and treat the recognized disease based almost exclusively on pharmacology and/or surgery.

It is also unfortunate that most hospitals and clinics, both public and private in many countries, do not consider the figure of the nutrition professional within the health team that cares for hospitalized patients, nor for those who are treated on an outpatient basis in specialized medical consultations. And it is for this reason that the nutritional aspect of a patient remains *orphaned* in most cases because the conventional medical system has separated it from the person, divorcing it from them in a radical and cruel way.

In truth, it can be said that there is an unbridgeable chasm between the conventional doctor's thinking and the nutritional aspects of a person, and this reality is detrimental to the patient, because, as has been demonstrated in this clinical case, if they had not been having made the necessary nutritional changes, Silvia would never have achieved the improvement she obtained, as in fact occurred for an entire year, when she was only treated with anti-inflammatories and methotrexate by the rheumatologist who treated her during that time.

When we look back at the historical past of medicine, from ancient Greece, Egypt, and Rome, the Arab world, the Renaissance and up to the 19th century, before the industrial revolution, the nutritional aspects of the patient were of vital importance for the doctor, who was also well versed in food and nutrition.

Let us remember the famous phrase of Hippocrates, father of Western medicine: *"Let your food be your medicine and your medicine be your food"*, which dates back to 450 BC, or the so-called healing power of food, a ardently belief defended and spread by famous doctors such as Avicenna and Maimonides in the 10th century, Paracelsus in the 16th century, Sebastian Kneipp, father of hydrotherapy and Samuel Hanneman, father of Homeopathy, in the 19th century.

Already in the 20th century and using the scientific method as a fundamental tool that guarantees the scientific aspect of a research, countless medical and nutritional articles have been published in prestigious journals, which reveal the works, which in this field of nutrition and disease, have been carried out in many universities and hospitals around the globe. There are also hundreds or thousands of books and magazines that illustrate this unavoidable relationship between health, illness, and nutrition.

One might then ask:

a.-At what point in the history of medicine, did the nutritional aspect of the patient stop being important for the doctor treating him?

b.-When and why did doctors stop studying nutrition during their university training?

c.-Why do doctors of the 20th century and those of the 21st century leave universities being very *ignorant* in matters of nutrition?

d.-Why do most conventional doctors view their patient's nutritional aspects with contempt and disqualification and in most cases leave them in a tunnel of darkness regarding what they should or should not eat, to recover from their illness?

e.-Why has current conventional medicine, and doctors trained under its criteria and doctrines, become blind, deaf, and dumb regarding the issue of nutrition and its relationship with health and illness, until to such an extent that it ignores, with arrogance, everything that is published, with a scientific nature, on this matter?

Surely, the answer to all these questions will be found in the so-called *Golden Age of Science, Medicine, and Chemistry*, specifically in the second half of the 19th century, when the so-called *Industrial Revolution* took place, which marked the birth of Pharmacology and the Pharmacological Industry.

This industry accumulated so much power that in a few years it invaded the world of medicine, the universities where doctors were trained, the hospitals where patients were treated, the laboratories where scientific research was carried out to validate and create the truths that supported medical practice, and finally all local medical associations and organizations, such as Medical Colleges and internationally, such as the World Health Organization.

In this way, it was able to consolidate in just 150 years of history what could be called a true *Medical Dictatorship*, which controls what is written, published, believed, rejected, studied, said, to the point of dictating what is true or false in matters of medicine; with the sole purpose of safeguarding its main interest, which is none other than financial interest and the accumulation of capital and power to unimaginable levels.

Chapter 13

Joan has chronic lumbago.

Joan is a 31-year-old nurse, who suffered from chronic low back pain since she was 24 years old, with 2 to 3 sciatica attacks per year. At the age of 25, she had an MRI of the entire spine, and they detected rectification of the cervical spine and intervertebral disc disease (*Discopathy*) at the lumbar level, in 3 places: L3-L4, L4-L5, L5- S1.

Joan is monitored by Traumatology, where she has been given treatment based on rest, painkillers, and aquatic physiotherapy to calm the painful crises. Her lumbago has worsened during 2017 and between March and April she suffered two muscle tears, in her back and left thigh, which is why she was prescribed treatment and rehabilitation, leaving her unable to work as an emergency medical nurse.

In the second half of 2017, Joan had a very poor quality of life, she lived with a constant tingling sensation in her back and left leg, she could not walk or stand for many hours, she did not drive her car and she could not do any type of exercise, which is why she gained 15 kilos in weight and felt worse. Being desperate about her situation, she decided to seek a second opinion and that is how she came to my office, hoping to find a solution to her medical condition.

What does Conventional Medicine think?

Disc disease is the most common disease of the spine, and it affects the intervertebral disc, is usually degenerative and associated with osteoarthritis.

Discopathy is the consequence of stiffness, dryness, and a progressive crushing of the intervertebral disc, very often the one located at the lumbosacral junction, in the L5 and S1 vertebrae, although this process appears at any level of the spinal column it can occur at any age, although aging favors it.

The disease is usually related to repeated microtrauma or physical stress, although it can also be due to congenital anomalies. It is very common to have osteoarthritis, a chronic disease that is manifested by persistent pain in the joints, caused by abnormal wear of the cartilage and the joint.

Generally, low back pain is the most common symptom. The progression of disc disease can also cause compression of the nerve roots, causing decreased sensitivity, tingling, a feeling of weakness and even pain in the legs, known as sciatica.

The best way to prevent disc disease is to do enough sports to ensure good back muscles to ensure better support, as well as a correct lifestyle to ensure good blood circulation. Losing weight may be necessary to lighten the load on the vertebrae, especially those in the lower back.

The diagnosis is made with the patient's history, with x-rays, and in some cases, with magnetic resonance imaging, which shows the degree of dehydration of the disc responsible for the impingement.

The treatment consists of relieving pain with the help of analgesics and anti-inflammatories, and for the same purpose, rehabilitation sessions can also be prescribed. These treatments combined with rest allow, in most cases, progressive relief to patients. Surgical intervention may be considered when pain is significant, when pharmacological treatments become ineffective, and when the disease causes neurological disorders such as motor deficits or sensory alterations.

What does non-conventional medicine think?

It is important to consider the participation of certain micronutrients in the treatment of disc disease and its complications.

*-Vitamin D deficiency:

Vitamin D deficiency, called hypovitaminosis, can affect men and women throughout life. This fat-soluble vitamin affects mineral metabolism and many other physiological functions. Hypovitaminosis D can result from several causes, such as poor vitamin D production in the skin due to lack of sun exposure, lack of dietary intake, accelerated losses of vitamin D, poor activation of vitamin D, and resistance to biological effects of active vitamin D.

Regardless of the cause, the manifestations of vitamin D deficiency are mainly due to impaired intestinal calcium absorption. Mild to moderate deficiency is usually asymptomatic.

Chronic deficiency causes hypocalcemia which can lead to secondary hyperparathyroidism and impaired skeletal mineralization, leading to osteopenia and decreased bone mineral density on radiographs.

Muscle pain is also possible and there is an increased risk of muscle tear occurring. Vitamin D deficiency in children can manifest as rickets, which is characterized by bowing of the legs. In adults, it is a cause of osteomalacia, and can promote osteoarthritis, due to poor mineralization of cartilage and bones. These disorders usually cause chronic muscle pain and discomfort, as well as fatigue, bone pain and generalized weakness.

Treatment of vitamin D deficiency should target the underlying disorder, if possible, and should also be tailored to the severity of the condition. Vitamin D replacement should always occur with calcium supplements because most of the harmful effects of vitamin D deficiency are due to disruptions of normal mineral ion homeostasis.

Encourage patients to consume foods rich in vitamin D, such as wild or canned salmon, cod liver oil, mackerel, pickled herring, and sun-dried shiitake mushrooms, and fortified foods such as milk, orange juice, yogurt, and margarine. Vitamin D produced in the skin because of sun exposure can last twice as long in the blood compared to ingested vitamin D. UV-B therapy has demonstrated greater efficacy in raising serum calcitriol levels compared to ingestion of a daily vitamin D 3 supplement.

*-Vitamin B12 deficiency:

Vitamin B12 is necessary to produce an adequate number of healthy red blood cells in the bone marrow. Vitamin B12 is available only in foods of animal origin (meat and dairy products) or yeast extracts (such as brewer's yeast). Vitamin B12 deficiency is defined by low levels of B12 stored in the body that can lead to anemia.

Vitamin B12 deficiency can develop for the following reasons:

.-Absence of intrinsic factor, also called pernicious anemia

.-Removal or destruction of the stomach

.-Excessive growth of bacteria in the small intestine (SIBO)

.-Dietary deficiency

Symptoms of hypovitaminosis B12 tend to develop slowly and may not be recognized immediately. As the condition worsens, common symptoms include:

- Weakness and fatigue
- Lightheadedness and dizziness
- Palpitations and rapid heartbeat.
- Difficulty breathing
- A sore tongue that has a red, fleshy appearance.
- Nausea or lack of appetite
- Weight loss
- Diarrhea
- Yellowish tint to the skin and eyes

If low B12 levels remain for a long time, the condition can also lead to irreversible damage to nerve cells, which can cause the following symptoms:

Numbness and tingling in hands and feet.
- Difficulty to walk
- Muscular weakness
- Irritability
- Memory loss

- Dementia
- Depression
- Psychosis

Treatment for this condition involves replacing the missing vitamin B12. People who cannot absorb B12 need regular injections. When injections are first given, a patient with severe symptoms may receive five to seven during the first week to restore the body's stores of this nutrient.

Acupuncture is effective in treating lower back pain. To reach this conclusion, the researchers recruited 143 patients with chronic low back pain who participated in a standard rehabilitation program, randomly half of the group also received two acupuncture sessions a week for three months. To make the comparison, participants answered a questionnaire before and after starting treatment, as well as three months after completing the study about quality of life and clinical data. At the end of the research, it was found that among the participants in the group that received acupuncture sessions there was a significantly greater improvement in quality of life, vitality, and mobility, compared to those who only participated in standard rehabilitation. Additionally, patients in the acupuncture group reported that pain while sitting, standing, as well as tingling in the hands and feet had decreased.

What was the treatment received by Joan?

When investigating Joan's eating habits, it caught our attention that she had a very unbalanced diet, with excessive consumption of:

*-Mineral thieves: red meats, simple sugars, refined flours, carbonated drinks, and coffee.

*-Milk and dairy derivatives: cheeses, butter, yogurts, kefir, creams

*-Sausages: sausage, salchichón, hams, mortadella, and chorizos

*-Candy: pastries and chocolate

In view of this, we performed a detailed clinical evaluation, added to laboratory tests, obtaining the following alterations:

*I was 15kg overweight

* Her left leg reflexes were diminished

* Raising her left leg woke her up with lower back pain

* Her back and leg muscles were very tender.

*She had decreased levels of vitamin B12, D3, iron and ferritin

*Her MRI showed disc disease between L4-L5, with degenerative changes, without having a herniated disc.

*Electromyography reflected chronic compression of the nerve root at L5, with muscle weakness in the left leg.

We propose that the combination of an acidifying diet, excess mineral thieves and hypovitaminosis D and B for years led Joan to suffer a weakening of her musculoskeletal system, to the point of suffering spontaneous muscle tears and with regular daily activity. For this reason, we set ourselves as our first objective the nutritional recovery of Joan for a period of 6 months and to observe the evolution of her symptoms.

The treatment consisted of:

a.-Nutritional support: basic rules of nutritional education were given.

.-Do not combine animal proteins with carbohydrates

.-Do not mix fruits with meals

.-Do not drink any drink with meals

.-Avoid red meat, and substitute white meat and fish

.-Eat more vegetable protein based on soy and other legumes

.-Increase fruits, vegetables, various seeds and nuts

.-Abolish the consumption of caffeinated drinks and soft drinks

.-Replace milk with coconut, oatmeal and rice vegetable drinks

b.-Nutritional supplementation: nutrients were supplied in high doses to recover vitamin and mineral deficiencies

• Group B vitamin complex intravenously

- Complex of minerals and trace elements intravenously
- Oral vitamin D3 and K2 in high doses: 10,000 IU and 100 mg/d
- Vitamin C at a dose of 5 grams intravenously
- Intravenous glutathione and lysine every other week

c.-Management of low back pain and generalized myalgia

- Acupuncture: one weekly session
- Magnetotherapy: one weekly session
- Laser therapy: one weekly session

After 3 months of taking this treatment regimen, Joan showed a progressive improvement in all her symptoms and her quality of life improved. She began to walk for longer, drive the car, and visit the gym once a week.

The treatment was spaced to biweekly sessions for another 3 months and at the end of six months, Joan fully recovered. All her laboratory tests were normalized, her lower back pain, the constant tingling sensation in her back, the weakness of her left leg disappeared, and she also lost 10kg of weight.

Joan returned to work as an emergency medical nurse after six months of treatment and was followed up with quarterly check-ups, checking the stability of her symptoms. She suspended her rehabilitation sessions and spaced her trauma consultations to every six months. By November 2019, Joan was still stable, and we discharged her from the clinic.

Conclusion and Discussion

Nutritional deficiencies represent another chapter of conventional medicine marked by *orphanhood and abandonment*, since no one wants them, because they arouse very little interest for most doctors in almost all specialties and for that reason, they are almost never thought in them, they are not investigated, they are not considered at all and are little treated by the average doctor.

Multiple nutritional deficiencies are responsible for a varied number of signs and symptoms that make up the so-called functional disease.

An imbalance that occurs in many organs and tissues due to the alteration of their normal functioning because of not having the biochemical elements necessary to fulfill their functions with their physiology in optimal shape. Because these symptoms do not represent a major alarm at first, most people ignore them, or at best silence them, self-medicating any symptom-suppressing medicine.

When a patient consults his primary care physician due to any symptoms of functional illness, he performs multiple examinations in search of a real illness to place the appropriate label, called a diagnosis, and then indicate the pharmacological or surgical treatment required, as established by an accepted protocol.

However, because functional disease is almost never detected by conventional medical analyzes and tests, since there is still no demonstrable lesion that can be revealed, the doctor, who is baffled by not being able to place the diagnostic label on the patient, ends up indicating an endless number of medications to treat the symptoms that disturb him, and when these treatments are not effective in solving the problem, which happens with a very high frequency, the doctor ends up referring the patient to another specialist, who almost it always ends up being the psychiatrist. This is the chain of events that occur with functionally ill people, and it is the reason why many of them are taking tranquilizers, anxiolytics, or antidepressants.

When the functional disease persists for a long period of time and is not treated effectively in its early stages, it can cause true organic damage in those tissues affected by a nutritional deficiency or a chronic accumulation of toxins, leading to many times to be irreversible.

At this time, the functional disease has evolved to injury disease, which can already be detected by laboratory tests, imaging techniques or invasive studies.

Conventional medicine is designed to detect the injury disease, diagnose it, and treat it with medications, surgery, laser, cryotherapy, etc.

It is therefore a fundamentally curative medicine, which acts in the final phase of the disease and does not have the capacity to detect it in its initial stage, much less prevent it.

Joan's experience clearly illustrates this line of thinking. She had been suffering from a clinical picture of low back pain for 7 years, starting at the age of 24. During all that time she probably ignored the symptom or silenced it with common painkillers. She consulted her primary care physician who performed a lumbar x-ray and, as no alteration was evident, she continued to recommend symptomatic medication and home rest. Already at the age of 31, when attacks of low back pain were frequent and disabling and associated with mild spontaneous muscle tears, her primary doctor referred her to the Traumatology service. There she was ordered to have an MRI of the spine and it was then that the degenerative disc disease was evident, requiring medication for chronic pain, rehabilitation, aquatic physiotherapy, and even temporary disability from work.

At no time during those 7 years did her treating doctor consider the possibility that the cause of the symptoms reported by Joan could be related to a chronic nutritional deficiency, specifically vitamin D3, B12, minerals and other micronutrients.

It is obvious that he also did not consider the possibility of recommending acupuncture and laser therapy to treat the low back pain attacks that she suffered. This therapeutic behavior cannot be expected from doctors, simply because it does not exist in their thinking, since they are not part of the paradigm of conventional medicine.

Chapter 14

Víctor has dizziness and a slow pulse.

When Víctor, a 45-year-old police officer, visited me in May 2015, he had been suffering for 8 months from frequent dizziness, sometimes accompanied by temporary fainting, which left him sweaty and feeling short of breath. He thought that these episodes were due to the excess stress that he always had at work, however, when he began to feel frequent episodes of palpitations and tachycardia, he decided to consult a cardiologist. The doctor placed a device on him for 24 hours to record the electrical activity of the heart, called arrhythmia Holter. Since this study showed that Víctor had a slow heart, with an average rhythm of 57 beats/minute, and a minimum of up to 32 beats/minute, lasting 14 hours, the cardiologist informed him that he should install a permanent Holter monitor, under the skin, in the chest, to record the electrical activity of his heart and decide if he was a candidate for a permanent pacemaker.

Víctor visited the cardiologist every month for a permanent arrhythmia Holter check, and in the first 2 months they had observed different types of alterations, although they were transitory and did not cause symptoms. Faced with the possibility of having to take heart medication for life, or worse yet, having to get a pacemaker, Víctor decided to seek a second opinion, and with that concern he came to my medical consultation.

What does Conventional Medicine think?

Heart rhythm problems, called *cardiac arrhythmia*, occur when the electrical impulses that coordinate the heartbeat do not work properly.

Your heart may beat too fast, too slow, or irregularly. Cardiac arrhythmias can cause you to have a fluttering sensation in your chest or a racing heart, and they can be harmless. However, some cardiac arrhythmias can cause bothersome and sometimes fatal signs and symptoms.

Although a heart rate less than 60 beats per minute is considered bradycardia, or a slow heart, it does not always indicate a problem. If you are physically fit, you may have an efficient heart capable of pumping an adequate supply of blood at less than 60 beats per minute at rest. Additionally, certain medications used to treat other conditions, such as high blood pressure, can slow your heart rate. However, if you have a slow heart rate and your heart is not pumping enough blood, you may have some symptoms.

Arrhythmias can make you feel premature heartbeats or feel like your heart is beating too slowly. Other signs and symptoms may be related to the heart not pumping effectively due to fast or slow heartbeats. These include shortness of breath, weakness, dizziness, lightheadedness, fainting or near-fainting, and chest pain or discomfort. Seek urgent medical attention if you experience any of these signs and symptoms suddenly or frequently, at a time when you would not expect to experience them.

There are a series of conditions or aspects of a person's lifestyle, in addition to some diseases, that can predispose to the development of a cardiac arrhythmia. Among the most common conditions, we have the following:

*Stress and anxiety

*Medicines

*Drink too much alcohol

*Caffeine, nicotine, or illegal drug use.

*Imbalance of minerals and electrolytes

*Obstructive sleep apnea

*Thyroid problems

*Mellitus diabetes

*High blood pressure

*Coronary artery disease,

*Congenital heart disease

*-Other heart problems and previous heart surgery

Cardiac arrhythmias can cause serious complications if they are not treated correctly and in a timely manner, for example:

*- They are associated with an increased risk of blood clots. If a clot breaks loose, it can travel from the heart to the brain. There it could block blood flow and cause a stroke.

*- Heart failure is a condition that can result if your heart is pumping ineffectively for a prolonged period due to bradycardia or tachycardia.

*-Some so-called malignant arrhythmias can cause the death of the person, without warning, in a case of sudden death.

The study of cardiac arrhythmia includes carrying out different types of evaluations, many of which require special equipment, such as:

*-Electrocardiogram

*-Portable 24-hour Holter recorder

*-Permanent implantable Holter recorder

*-Heart ultrasound

*-Stress test

*-Electrophysiological tests

Treatment of cardiac arrhythmia will depend on its type and severity, and may include the following:

*-Antiarrhythmic medications

*-Electrical cardioversion

*-Catheter ablation inside the heart

*-Pacemaker and/or implantable automatic defibrillator (ICD)

*-Surgery for some cases.

What does non-conventional medicine think?

To prevent cardiac arrhythmia, it is important to lead a heart-healthy lifestyle to reduce the risk of heart disease. A heart-healthy lifestyle may include the following:

*-Consume a heart-healthy diet

*-Stay physically active and maintain a healthy weight

*-Avoid smoking

*-Limit or avoid caffeine and alcohol

*-Reduce intense stress and anger

*-Use over-the-counter medications with caution, as some cold and cough medications contain stimulants that can trigger a rapid heartbeat.

You can stop an arrhythmia that begins in the upper chambers of the heart by using so-called vagal maneuvers that include, holding your breath and pressing, dipping your face in ice water or coughing. These maneuvers affect the nervous system that controls the heartbeat (*vagus nerves*), often causing the heart rate to slow down. However, they do not work for all types of arrhythmias.

There is extensive literature that supports the use of micronutrients to help prevent and even treat some types of arrhythmias. The best known are:

a.-Magnesium:

The effectiveness of magnesium administration in the control of cardiac arrhythmias has been established in the last 50 years, but until the early 1970s it was not demonstrated that its effect is due to the correction of a pre-existing magnesium deficiency rather than the therapeutic role of a high magnesium intake. Magnesium has also given good results in those cases that do not respond completely or are refractory to conventional treatment.

b.-Potassium:

Potassium is the most abundant intracellular cation. The proportion between intracellular and extracellular potassium is one of the factors that most influences the conduction of nerve impulses and the contraction of muscle cells, including myocardial cells. Therefore, small alterations in its concentrations can cause severe symptoms at the level of the electrical rhythm of the heart.

c.-Calcium:

Recently there is much interest in cellular abnormalities of calcium homeostasis in the human heart. For this reason, it is equally important to monitor blood calcium levels in case of cardiac arrhythmia. Intravenous calcium can slow the heart rate and has been used in the treatment of tachycardia.

d.-Zinc:

Although research in humans is still in its infancy, there is evidence that zinc supplements protect the heart from arrhythmias and stroke, in rats and mice. What's more, there is a clinical study that found that heart failure is closely related to zinc deficiency. Another study showed that high doses can prevent and treating angina and arrhythmias in patients with atherosclerosis.

e.-Coenzyme Q10:

Improving cardiac strength is exactly what Q10 offers cardiac patients. Heart failure is a condition in which the heart lacks the strength to pump blood to all parts of the body and is a common cause of cardiac arrhythmia.

f.-Taurine:

It is an amino acid that can help reduce the risk of cardiovascular disease. Research shows a link between high levels of taurine and significantly lower rates of mortality related to heart disease, as well as reductions in blood pressure and cardiac arrhythmias.

g.-Carnitine:

It is an amino acid that is linked to improvements in patients with serious heart disorders, such as coronary heart disease, chronic heart failure, and cardiac arrhythmias. A 12-month study noted a reduction in heart failure and deaths among participants who took L-carnitine supplements.

What was the treatment followed by Victor?

Victor was instructed to follow a treatment plan based on three aspects:

a.-Lifestyle:

*-Eliminate smoking

*-Eliminate stimulating drinks such as tea, coffee, etc.

*-Eliminate alcohol in all its forms

*-Change jobs and reduce or eliminate stress

*-Do moderate and regular aerobic physical exercise.

b.-Heart-healthy diet

*-Increase the consumption of fruits, vegetables, and greens

*-Increase the consumption of legumes and nuts

*-Consume 3 daily servings of whole grains

*-Ingest 3 raw tablespoons of extra virgin vegetable oil (olive, coconut)

*-Consume blue fish (sardine, tuna, salmon, mackerel, dogfish) at list 100 to 150 grams 3 times a week.

*-Avoid trans fats, red meat, sausages, milk and derivatives, refined salt, and sugar.

c.-Cardiohealthy Supplementation

.-Potassium, zinc and magnesium; regulate heart rate

.-Selenium and germanium; they are antioxidants

.-Vitamin A, C, E: they are natural antioxidants

.-Coenzyme Q10; improves the energy performance of the heart

.-Taurine; helps regulate blood pressure and heart rate

.-Carnitine; improves the energy performance of the heart

How did Victor evolve?

Víctor was evaluated every 3 months to verify that he complied with all the recommendations for lifestyle, diet and heart-healthy supplementation, and to evaluate the cardiology notes on the review of the content of the Holter recorder every month, the result of his laboratory tests every six months and tolerance to the treatment provided. The results observed were the following:

*-The episodes of arrhythmia were spaced out over time until they disappeared almost completely in the first year

*-The most lasting arrhythmia was sinus bradycardia, with cardiac pauses or stops of up to 3 seconds.

*-After 5 years of follow-up, the use of pharmacological medication to control the arrhythmia has not been necessary

*-The placement of a pacemaker has also not been required since the pauses or stops have disappeared in the last year.

*-The patient has maintained his heart-healthy lifestyle and has enjoyed a good level and quality of life.

Conclusions and Discussion

There is extensive literature, of scientific publications, in many prestigious medical journals, related to the beneficial effect that some natural supplements have on the control and regulation of heart rate, to the point that statements such as this have been published:

"It is preferable to restore normal magnesium levels in the body before instituting antiarrhythmic medications. No cardiac arrhythmia should be considered refractory before considering magnesium supplementation, as well as other electrolytes such as potassium, calcium, zinc, etc." (Lancet, Sep 1991).

However, the use of cardio regulatory minerals, cardio energetic amino acids, cardiotonic vitamins or natural antioxidants does not exist and are not used by conventional cardiologists, and furthermore, they are rejected or simply disqualified with phrases such as: " *all these remedies are placebo"*, *"There is no publication that demonstrates its effectiveness,"* *"these supplements cannot be compared with the high potency and effectiveness of the medications."*

Most conventional doctors of all specialties, including cardiologists, are unaware that there are medical master's courses in the field of *Integrative Medicine, Functional Medicine, or Systemic Medicine,* which are taught by world-renowned universities such as Stanford, Harvard or Yale, and that enjoy acceptance and recognition by the international medical community.

From the practice of these new modalities of medicine, the use of natural remedies, orthomolecular supplements, medicinal plants, and nutritional measures is supported and considered to treat many diseases, either in unique schemes or complementing conventional pharmacological schemes.

Medicine in the new millennium is changing slowly and progressively and is moving towards the integration and synergy of all types of treatments and therapies, natural or not, based on scientific evidence and supported by publications that demonstrate their effectiveness and safety. More and more patients are seeking this type of integrative approach and in a few decades, the conventional medical community will have to evolve towards this integration, or it will simply fall further and further behind, in the corner of oblivion, until it reaches its minimum expression and even become extinct.

Epilogue

Final thoughts

Dear reader, I can assure you that during my extensive medical experience of more than 37 years until today, I have witnessed hundreds or thousands of cases of patients who have had experiences like the ones I have shared with you in this book, and I have not incorporated them here because I would need to write many books to capture them and because I don't want to abuse your patience and bore you with such a long story. However, I have shown you the story lived by 14 people who came to my office with their unresolved health problems, with the hope of finding a solution and breaking the chains of failure, frustration, and hopelessness that their treating doctors had left them previous; and I consider that all the information contained in those 14 stories is sufficient to support the message that I wish to convey through my words, which spring from a professional life dedicated to medicine.

To conclude this story, here in its epilogue, I cannot say goodbye without leaving my final reflections for all the patients and brave readers who have had the courage to reach this point in their reading, and I want to warn you that it is possible that when as you read these final reflections, you will experience different emotions that can be good or bad, depending on which part of your ego they awaken. In any case, I want to offer you my most sincere apologies, because it is not my intention to awaken negative emotions or make you have a bad time.

However, if my arguments have managed to generate a conflict within your soul, regarding the way you have lived the medicine, whether as a patient or as a doctor, I believe that my objective has been met.

To my readers who are healthy people, who have never had to seek a medical consultation and have never interacted with hospitals, clinics and laboratories, first of all I want to congratulate you because you belong to a privileged group of people who enjoy well-being and good health, the treasure most valuable thing we can possess, because without it, nothing in this world is possible.

My final thoughts for this class of readers is that they do everything possible to maintain their state of health and well-being, because to maintain this type of privilege you have to work and pay a price, you have to build a lifestyle that promotes and sustains that health condition, because otherwise, that state of well-being that you enjoy at this moment could collapse and transform into a state of a sick patient who must fight to return to the happy state of health that he had in the past.

Reading the stories of my 14 patients you were able to realize what their lives were like as patients, the reasons why they reached that state, everything they struggled with official medicine, for years, even running serious dangers that could have cost them their lives. You also witnessed their impressive changes when they decided, bravely, often against the opinion of friends, family, and health professionals, to follow a different path, most of the time overwhelmed and desperate by the suffering their illness caused them, and that is how they managed to regain their health and learn a lesson that changed their lives forever.

I invite you, my healthy reader, to see these 14 stories as a movie that is showing you what could happen to you if you were to change sides and therefore, learn from the message that arises from the struggle of each of those people to recover their health and apply it in your life and that of your loved ones so that they are always healthy people and never enter the territory of illness.

But since we cannot be eternal, it is possible that sooner or later you will receive the unexpected visit of an illness, which has come to stay in your life, temporarily or permanently, depending on how you treat it and who you are willing to do to get her out of your life. When that moment comes, which I hope will be very late, I ask you to remember this book and the story of my 14 patients, who wanted to convey this message to you, which I hope can be useful to you when it is your turn, as it will be the turn of all of us, be a patient.

To my readers who are sick people, that is, patients, as they are called in hospitals and in the health sector in general, the first thing I want to tell you is that I understand you, much more than you may think, basically because I have been through 37 years of my life speaking, knowing and helping thousands of patients to solve their health problems, and through that long experience I have been able to feel and see up close the thousand faces of the disease and the way it impacts the physical, mental, emotional, spiritual and social of each of the people who suffer from it. In addition to this, I want to tell you that I understand you even more, because I have also been a sick patient, and throughout my life I have faced gastritis, gastroesophageal reflux, hemorrhoids, urinary stones, an enlarged prostate, high blood pressure, and covid complicated with pneumonia.

So, I've been in those shoes, and I know exactly what it feels like. I have suffered the rigors of these illnesses; I have feared for my life and I have cried bitter tears when I have lost that precious treasure that is health.

My final reflections for you are to sigh and feel the strength of hope, because my 14 patients, whose experiences you have already read, just want to convey the message that there are solutions for diseases considered incurable by conventional medicine.

The message of hope is for each patient who suffers from a disease, whether they have it under control, and even more so if they have it uncontrolled and live devastated with terrible symptoms that cause them to have a very poor quality of life. The story of my 14 patients, which is the same story of hundreds and thousands of patients that I have known and cared for, what I want to convey to them is that there is hope and real possibilities to get out of the dark world of the disease and return to the bright world of health. If you have not found that change and that solution, which is what we long for when we are sick, then you already know that there are other paths, real, true, proven, recommended, and endorsed by many patients and many doctors around the world that we have chosen unconventional or traditional medicine, as the WHO calls it, and which is already in a phase of integration with official medicine, to provide the best solutions in the task of defeating diseases. Furthermore, if you still have doubts, holistic and integrative medicine is also supported by solid scientific evidence, you just must do a little research and you will see it.

The other final reflection I have for my dear sick patient readers is that you have immense power in your hands, which you must realize, to use it for the benefit of yourselves and for that of medicine as an institution. You make up a gigantic conglomerate around the world and represent a matrix force with great potential and if you direct that potential to influence the medical institution you could be the determining factor in rescuing it from the abyss into which it has fallen and returning it to the dignified and glorious role that it has always occupied in society, working tirelessly and with compassion for the well-being of humanity affected by the disease.

You, my dear sick patient readers, have the power in your hands to unleash the Great Medical Revolution of the 21st century, which can put an end to the abomination that official conventional medicine has been practicing and give way to the growth of a truly humanized medicine that is efficient and compassionate with suffering humanity. And you don't have to be surprised by this idea, because you don't have to do anything extraordinary, even if the word revolution sounds like conflict and inspires fear in you. You just must find out what your rights are as a patient, which are established and inscribed in the

Universal Declaration of Patients' Rights, issued in the last third of the 20th century, and which you can surely find in any internet search engine, such as Google or Yahoo, for example.

If each patient, fully aware of their rights, begins to demand that they be fulfilled by each of the doctors who care for them in any hospital, health center, medical center, outpatient clinic or private clinic, I can assure you that they will generate an immense pressure and a gigantic conflict within the heart of conventional medicine. Which by not being able to give a coherent answer to the problem, because it does not have one, will end up suffering a fatal heart attack.

When you know your rights as a patient and decide to start fighting, with bravery, determination and courage, to defend them in all areas, aware that you are risking your health and your life, or that of your loved ones who may also be sick patients in this moment; you will be able to have precise and clear ideas and arguments to talk to your doctor, and every time you feel that he is acting in favor of other interests and turning his back on your interests, which should be the only ones to which he should be devoted, you will be able to rebuke him. and invite you to reflect.

To do that, you will only have to look him directly in the eyes, knowing that this professional has, or is supposed to have, a vocation in his heart that prompted him to study medicine for a long time and with great sacrifice he finished his career and surely after he did one or several specialties, with a lot of work and sacrifice as well, and you will tell him in your own words, something like this:

"Doctor, with all the gratitude that I profess to you for what you have done and continue to do for me, and with all the respect that you deserve for your training and professional practice, I must tell you something that I hope does not make you feel offended or disrespected, because that is not my intention, and if you should feel that way, I beg you, with all my heart, to forgive me.

What I want to tell you is that I feel that you are not complying with my rights as a patient and you are failing in your sacred vocation as a doctor, the one that has led you to study and work with sacrifice for so many years to get here, just to be in front of to one more patient that is me; and I say this, because I do not feel satisfied with your assistance, because you have not shown commitment, respect and compassion in the resolution of my health problem, because you do not dedicate time to me, because you do not talk to me to explain to me what I have, the pros and the cons of the treatments that you has sent me, the other treatment possibilities that exist, because you have not shown me your determination to break all the prejudices and go as far as you have to go to help me recover my health, which I have lost, and remains in the condition of a suffering patient. On the contrary, you have limited yourself to seeing me as just another patient, to whom you dedicate the minimum necessary, following an institutional protocol, without leaving your comfort zone and ensuring your financial profitability above all, and as a consequence of this, I continue to be a slave to pharmacies, hospitals, and laboratories, to live in a dark tunnel of insecurity, unhappiness and suffering, enduring the rigors of an illness that you have not been able to overcome, because you have called it incurable, idiopathic, of unknown cause or any other argument that explains its inability to resolve it. I would love for you tonight, when you put your head on your pillow, to think about my words and ask yourself this question: at what point did I lose the true essence of being a doctor? And if you manage to answer it, I hope that when you wake up the next morning, you get out of bed with the determination to begin to rescue yourself as a professional and once again place your humble patients, like me, in the priority of your medical act."

To my readers who are medical students, who spend most of their days at the Faculty of Medicine, studying to become the next generation of relief doctors.

Those who will be the future directors of hospitals, ministers of health, heads of groups research, heads of some specialized medical department or epidemiologists and public health workers. Or simply doctors dedicated to running their private or hospital practice, living thousands of experiences with their patients, in other words, those they have in their hands, in this moment, what will be the future of medicine. For you I also have some final thoughts.

Surely if you bought this book, it was because the title caught your attention, or the description of it that I wrote on the back cover. That Second Opinion phrase or the other Alternative Solution phrase may have resonated with something that you carry in your heart or deep in your mind, and perhaps that is a sign that indicates that you are a good candidate to explore and perhaps study at some point in your future, everything that so-called other medicine, also known as traditional, integrative or biological, has to offer you. I do not rule out that a few other medical students who have this book in their hands may have done so on the recommendation of another, because it was given to them as a gift or because they bought it out of curiosity, but the majority of these students will have immediately ruled me out upon reading the description of it or perhaps they reached the prologue, and thought of yet another charlatan, and threw the book anywhere, if not the trash can. These types of students do not waste their time reading what they consider pseudoscientific garbage, which is the favorite derogatory phrase of their medical professors to refer to everything that has to do with the world of unconventional medicine, because these types of students of medicine, are those who have suffered most intensely from the indoctrination of deification that is suffered in medical school.

My first reflection for my dear medical student readers, regardless of their category, who have had the experience of reading the entire content of this book and have reached this point, is a kind of warning about which I want to warn you. When you began medical studies, you began a project that would last between 5 and 8 years, depending on the country where you are studying, and during that time you will live or suffer, an indoctrination process of deification with almost religious and fundamentalist features, of the which almost no one will notice.

The indoctrination process of deification will transform them into a different person than the one they were when they began their studies, their vision of the world, of society and of people will change, and as their knowledge increases and they pass subjects and moving from one year to the next, they will feel in the depths of their subconscious that they belong to a privileged class of person who is being given special knowledge with great power to influence the lives of all their future patients, to eradicate their illnesses and diseases, understand their behaviors and affect their decisions. This power will give them an extraordinary feeling of superiority, invested with a strong load of arrogance, all supported by a floor of arrogance that will be manifested in their verbal language and especially gestural.

At the end of the process, when they graduate as doctors, they will receive the title of gods of Olympus in the auditorium of their university, and then they will begin to practice in clinics and hospitals as true know-it-alls who walk on a red carpet all the time, and who see all the other beings that surround them, as of lesser human category, insignificant ignorant people who do not have the slightest idea of what the human body is.

How it works and how it relates to a society and an environment, which also they know it perfectly, and all that knowledge, which they acquired with so much study and sacrifice for more than five years, deserves to receive special and almost reverential treatment.

Deification indoctrination affects all medical students to a varying degree of intensity, depending on the previous values and principles that formed their personality before coming to medical school. This process is not a coincidence or something natural but is part of a well-studied and designed plan to turn them all into slaves and the best defenders of the conventional medical institution, as well as the perfect pawns of the pharmaceutical industry, the provider mother of all the financial resources that support the infrastructure on which most universities, hospitals, clinics, institutes, ministries of health operate and even the WHO. During the deification indoctrination process, great emphasis and importance is given to creating the mentality and conviction in the student, that he must see and perceive everything that comes from the so-called unconventional medicine, as pseudoscientific information that the only thing intended is it is swindling the unwary, ripping off its clients, and practicing the professional intrusion of sacrosanct conventional medicine, the only holder of scientific truth since it is fully accredited by all national and international institutions. For all this, future doctors must reject, disqualify, and discredit with all the force of their reason and their negative emotions all those who practice or sympathize with that world, whoever they may be, from simple general practitioners to Nobel Prize winners in medicine, which must be perceived as contaminated with the curses and intellectual garbage of a pagan pseudo-medicine.

Since I also spent 7 years in medical school, I also experienced that indoctrination of deification and that is why I can talk to you about it as I am doing, and not because I have read it in some magazine or book, but because I suffered it firsthand and I made many patients suffer through it during the first 15 years of my medical practice.

To give you an idea of the magnitude of the damage that this terrible indoctrination of deification can create in the doctor-patient relationship, I am going to inform you that in Spain, when you are going to register for the first time in the medical school to practice your profession, they demand a very curious requirement from you, you must acquire *Personal Protection Insurance*, something that I had never heard of in the previous 24 years that I worked between Venezuela and the United States. When I asked what that insurance consisted of and why I should take it, they responded that in Spain it is common for patients to attack doctors, and that they have even gone so far as to murder some doctors, due, most of the time, to alleged mistreatment and contempt on the part of the doctor and/or malpractice that affected seriously the health and life of a patient or some of their family members.

The second reflection I have for you, my dear medical student reader, is that not everything that glitters is gold. I want you to know that in 2000, as chief cardiologist at a district hospital in Venezuela, I was invited by the pharmaceutical industry to attend the world congress of cardiology sponsored by the American Heart Association (AHA), in the city of New Orleans.

I shared a week with more than 10,000 cardiologists from all over the world, concentrated in a Convention Center, a 5-story building with hundreds of luxurious rooms where more than 30 daily conferences were held simultaneously, with hotel, meals, books and magazines, everything. included and covered by the pharmaceutical industry. The interesting thing about the story is that on the last day of the event I attended a conference given by the president of the AHA of that year, and one of the most prominent cardiologists in the US at that time.

The title of his lecture was *Critical reading of scientific literature*, and the room was packed, with about 200 cardiologists in attendance. At that conference, this colleague said that we had to be very careful when we read the works published in scientific medical journals, whatever they were, because the reality is that more than 75% were *biased*.

Throughout the conference he presented more than 20 articles taken from journals such as Lancet, New England Journal of Medicine, JAMA, and many others considered serious and credible. He presented evidence of how the statistical information from more than 70% of the articles presented was manipulated to reach the articles' conclusions, which were all favorable to support the use of a new medication to treat various cardiovascular diseases. How statistics uses a very technical and hermetic language that most doctors do not understand, with rare exceptions, because that is the point where the pharmaceutical industry creates its great legal tricks to support the great lies that it sells to us as unquestionable and absolutely truths scientific, and all conventional doctors believe them as if they were teachings emanating from God.

Since the pharmaceutical industry controls the contents of what is taught in medical schools, I invite you to think about how many lies they will not be able to tell you in the years that you will be receiving your indoctrination of deification, and you believe them all, because that information it is backed by an entire university medical institution and by accredited doctors, who are your professors.

The main objective of scientific publications is to establish the scientific dogmas prevailing in each era of history, and thus, any prestigious magazine admits publishing a crazy work if it meets two conditions:

That it sounds good and that it supports the prejudices of the editors. Studies published by the magazines themselves, statements by their editors and an analysis of their relations with the pharmaceutical industry allow us to conclude that the manipulation and falsification of data, censorship and methodological and moral perversions are a structural problem derived from the function of science as a holder of power.

The evidence of this reality is overwhelming I can't write down all the references, because I would have to write another complete book for it, but I am going to give you some data, the veracity of which you can check whenever you want.

* -Dr. Jim Nuovo published an article in JAMA where he presents his conclusions from the review of 359 studies on new drugs published between 1989 and 1998 in prestigious journals such as Lancet, BMJ, JAMA, etc. Only 26 of them had published statistics that collected the

side effects of the treatments on the patients. That is, 333 studies lied or omitted data.

*-Richard Smith, the editor of BMJ, one of the most important magazines in the world, made one of the harshest statements that the scientific community can receive: *"Clinical research fraud is like child abuse, once it exists you are beginning to see how common it is."* The editor spoke these words during the celebration of the first international medical congress in Hong Kong. He insisted that both the detection and investigation methods, as well as the conclusions of clinical trials, are dishonest and completely inadequate. Fraud cases include fabrication of data or complete fabrication of data. This expert insisted on the need for institutions to create mechanisms to avoid this unethical behavior (El Mundo 12/13/98).

The average reader of scientific journals are health professionals and researchers in their multiple branches, and they believe that what they publish is real:

*-That knowing the human genome will allow us to eradicate diseases

*-That vaccines helped eradicate contagious diseases

*-That the only way to control HIV is with aggressive drugs

*-And a Long etc, etc, etc, etc.

What if most doctors suddenly became aware that the information, they receive is not the truth, the whole truth and nothing but the truth, but is produced by those who control these journals? What if decided to acknowledge that there are honest and independent scientists who offer alternative analyzes and results?

My third and final reflection for you, a medical student, is that you must be aware that you are the future of medicine and can play an important active role in the Great Medical Revolution of the 21st century.

And your role as a soldier in that battle it is to protect your purity and your potential, right now that you are training as a doctor. To achieve this, you must look for mechanisms to fight against the indoctrination of deification, such as seeking the help of a psychologist to allow you to detect traits of megalomania, self-sufficiency, and arrogance in your personality and give you tools to combat them, and you must do this from now and mainly after you graduate and start practicing. Another mission for this soldier is to question and not believe anything his teachers tell him or read in scientific journals, unless he compares the information with other media, such as non-conventional medical literature.

Only accept information in which there is no clue of the intervention of the pharmaceutical industry in that article, magazine, book or publishing institution, and discard everything published that does not have the authors' declaration that they do not incur conflicts of interest.

If you manage to leave medical school free of all these prejudices, which is going to cost you a lot of work, perhaps you can do your bit to rescue a more honest and humane medicine and save yourself from the clutches of medicine conventional that waits for you to become its slave and pawn so that you work tirelessly to increase their treasury coffers.

My last reflections are for my colleagues, practicing doctors, regardless of their status, generalists, specialists, or super specialists, from simple primary care doctors to the imminent chief doctors of hospitals, clinics, research groups, or professors. university students.

I am aware that most likely the number of conventional doctors who buy and read this book will be very low and poor, because perhaps, just upon reading the title they will be scared and not even touch it, much less skim it to see what it is about treats. Only the phrase Alternative Solution will trigger all the alarms that you carry in your brain and that were burned into you since your time as a medical student and continually reinforced in each refresher course, medical conference or master's or specialization course that you have taken since. having graduated from medical school.

As I also know that someone or another may buy and read this book, motivated by curiosity or perhaps because at some time, or recently, they have felt attracted to know a little more about non-conventional medicine, because some patients in their practice or than that of other colleagues, have reflected great improvements and even the total healing of a health disorder, after having been treated by a doctor of the other medicine and he or his colleagues had failed before with those patients, even after having applied the most innovative treatments recommended by the pharmaceutical industry and/or the articles published by the most famous scientific journals.

In any case, I trust that after reading this entire book, it can create at least a sense of internal conflict or increase the doubts that any conventional doctor may have, due to the results he has obtained in his medical practice, based 100% on the use of medications.

I am also aware that the reflections that I am going to offer to my colleagues, the conventional doctors, who have the strange and inexplicable experience of having read me completely, are going to collide resoundingly against the walls of solid stone that lie in their brains and sustained because of the deification indoctrination they received in medical school and have maintained over the years because it is an inherent part of their medical personality. My reflections will also crash against the million false data that my colleagues have stored in their memories after having received so much medical information from books, magazines, podcasts, conferences, master's, and postgraduate courses, all of which they have considered 100% true and scientific, without even suspecting that reality is totally different, as we have already demonstrated in the previous paragraphs.

However, if after having read this entire book, and especially my last reflections given in this epilogue, I manage to awaken, even in just one of them, a spark of light in their cerebral cortex or in their emotional brain, may I do so. think and/or feel, that perhaps I could be right and for that reason he himself has seen and verified how most of the patients he has treated throughout his medical career, with few exceptions, have never been completely healed of their chronic and degenerative diseases, having to settle for good control of the symptoms that overwhelm their patients even though to do so they have had to turn them into happy slaves of pharmacies, I would consider the mission that this publication pursues accomplished.

My first reflection for my medical readers, I am going to make them from the suffering and pain they have felt when they or a very dear family member have ever fallen ill in a worrying way.

When we doctors or a very close family member has fallen prey to a worrying illness, we usually look for the best of our medical colleagues to receive treatment, one with whom we can talk, who explains to us all the details, time and patience, who inspires confidence in us that it has been the best option we have chosen because he is very qualified, has had previous experiences in solving similar cases and will do everything possible, with ethics and commitment to solve our health problem.

Hippocrates in his famous oath states: *"Every doctor is obliged to treat each patient as if they were a very beloved family member, with the same dedication, commitment and love."*

So, I invite you to ask yourself if you practice this Hippocratic mandate in your consultation, or on the contrary, do you usually treat your patients from your usual deified indoctrination and treat them as inferior beings and yet, when it is you or a family member who is sick, you look for and want the best possible doctor.

If you are that type of doctor who uses that double standard, of giving the minimum of your professionalism to your patients, because you are not going to sacrifice your comfort zone, but you want the best of a colleague's professionalism when it comes to you or from a family member, then you are simply violating the Hippocratic command and you are betraying your vocation. That's why I invite you to reflect on it and every time you have a patient in front of you, think about your family member when they were very sick, all the anguish, despair and suffering you went through until the problem was overcome and put yourself in their shoes of your patient and feel sorry for him or her as much as you would for a sick family member.

My last reflection for you, my appreciated medical reader, is to incorporate you into the Great Medical Revolution of the 21st Century, an experiment that we must all execute together and at the same time, the general public, sick patients, medical students and practicing doctors in order to save to medicine, our beloved profession, from the clutches of the abomination of a criminal mafia that is using it for the sole purpose of excessive profit, crushing in the process everything that has been part of medicine for millennia: the patient-doctor relationship, the detailed questioning and physical examination, the freedom of the doctor to think, deduce and act based on the information that his patient has given him.

The right of both the doctor and the patient to choose the best possible treatment, whether conventional or unconventional, but with the assurance of scientific support that it will work optimally, and all framed in the respect, commitment, compassion, and ethics that we must maintain with each of the patients.

While medical students, patients and the public must take the rearguard of this revolution that aims to rescue 21st century medicine, we are the practicing doctors, those already graduated and with experience, who are called to be the soldiers that they must go to the front of this battle to fight it with our best weapons, those that we have developed throughout our professional experience, and that we wear with the symbol of a white coat, which represents our vocation and commitment.

It is not about going on medical strikes and paralyzing hospitals, nor marching with banners in front of pharmaceutical lobbies demanding improvements for us in our demands.

This is something different, deeper, and more intelligent that we must do to have a truly transformative effect on current medical practice.

What I suggest you do as a volunteer soldier in this battle for our medicine is a change of attitude on your part. On the one hand, try to fight against the indoctrination of deification that characterizes your medical personality in front of the patient, since you left medical school and that has surely increased over the years to the extent that you have acquired much more information through the courses, master's degrees and postgraduate degrees that you have taken, which far from making you more humble have brought you closer to the gods of Olympus, creating a great abyss of separation between you and your poor patients.

On the other hand, I suggest that you try to remove from your brain all the false information that you have accumulated over the years receiving medical information from a single sector, the pharmaceutical industry, whose veracity has been called into question, such as I mentioned in previous paragraphs, with overwhelming evidence demonstrated by two scientific works published in the same journals that they use to deceive you publication after publication. Try to contrast all the information you have by looking for different sources of information, you can start with the extensive bibliography that I present in this book, and I suggest that every time you go to treat a new patient you try to investigate what non-conventional medicine thinks regarding the origin, evolution and treatment of this pathology, and if you apply the best that your criteria indicate in order to offer the best of the two medicines to your patient, I assure you that you will begin to see the same results that I have described in the 14 clinical cases. And if you don't feel safe or confident using therapies that you don't know or master, simply try to train yourself in these new areas, in any of the universities and institutions that offer them, which now abound everywhere.

What I am suggesting to you is that you transform yourself into another kind of doctor, one who understands that medicine is a tool that only belongs to doctors and that we are formed with an ethical mandate to use it solely and exclusively to generate good for ourselves our patients and all of hurt humanity and never to harm them, as stated in the first and most radical of the Hippocratic principles: *First do no harm.*

If you continue to be the pawn of the pharmaceutical industry, which you surely are without knowing it, and you verify and reaffirm it every time you use your pen to write in your prescription the medications that you are going to recommend to your patient and to all of them, in each medical consultation, without caring what happens to that patient, without assessing the side effects, without knowing if their quality of life will improve or worsen or even if they could die as a consequence of the effects of that medication. If you continue down that path, without questioning anything the pharmaceutical industry tells you, while enjoying your comfort zone, you will be pushing our beloved medicine into the abyss into which it has been thrown by that criminal mafia that has parasitized it but that wants us deceive by presenting herself as the great benefactor of this story.

These reflections that I am offering you will only be able to gain fertile ground in your heart if you truly possess a true medical vocation and are not one of those cases who studied medicine for any other reason, such as a family pattern or the search for social prestige, or If you are not a doctor who studied this profession driven by a true vocation, but who has lost it or buried it somewhere along the path, to replace it with other values of a political, financial, administrative nature, etc., that better suit your needs interests and a wide comfort zone. But this analysis is not my responsibility to do, and it is something that only your own consciousness can do.

Chapter 1

1.-McNally EM, Kaltman JR, Benson DW, et al;Working Group of the National Heart, Lung, and Blood Institute; Parent Project Muscular Dystrophy. *Trastornos Cardiacos asociados a la Distrofia Muscular de Becker y Duchenne. Circulation.* 2015;131(18):1590-1598.

2.-McNally, Elizabeth M., MD. *Miocardiopatia en la Distrofia Muscular, ¿Cuándo tratar?.* The Journal of the American Medical Association (JAMA). Febrero 20, 2017.

3.- Bourke JP, Bueser T, Quinlivan R. *Prevención y tratamiento de las complicaciones cardíacas en la distrofia muscular de Duchenne y Becker y la miocardiopatía dilatada ligada al cromosoma X.* Octubre 2018. La Biblioteca Cochrane

4.-www.ornish.com : 37 años de evidencia científica por Dean Ornish, MD® 2019

5.-The HALE project, JAMA 292: 1433-1439, 2004. Mediterranean diet and CAD.

6.-J Am Coll Cardiol 45: 1379-1387, 2005. Diet and cardiovascular disease

7.-JAMA 288: 2569-2578, 2002. Optimal diets for prevention of CAD

8.-Circulation 99: 779-785, 1999. Mediterranean diet after Miocardial Infarction

9.-JAMA 292: 1440-1446, 2004. Mediterranean diet and endothelian dysfunction

10.-JAMA 293: 43-53, 2005. Comparison Ornish, Atkins, Zone diet and CAD

11.-Lancet 343: 807-809, 1994. Magnesium and Myocardial Infarction

12.-Circulation 92: 2617-2621, 1995. Magnesium reduce MI size

13.-Biomed Environ Sci 10: 220-226, 1997. Selenium and cardiovascular disease

14.-Acta Diabetol 37: 33-39, 2000. Niacina y Peroxidación lipídica

15.-J Clin Endocrinol Metabol 86: 1845-1846, 2001. Homocysteine, B9 y B12 vitamin

16.-Circulation 97: 2222-2229, 1998. Vit C improves endothelium function

17.-Clin Science 98: 455-460. Vit C improves CV response in smokers

18.-Am Heart J 97: 378-388, 1979. Role of L-Carnitine in fatty acid metabolism on ischemic myocardium

19.-Clin Cardiol 8: 267-282, 1985. Therapeutic effect of taurine in CHF

Chapter 2

1.-Cañate, Jorge, MD y Arequipa M. Adrian Arturo. *Tejido Linfoide Asociado a Mucosas : MALT, GALT, BALT, SALT.* Universidad Técnica de Manabi, Cátedra de Inmunología. Enero 2020. https://www.slideshare.net/adriancitoarequipa/malt-tejido-linfoide-asociado-a-mucosas

2.-Castrillón Rivera, Laura, et all. *La Función Inmunológica de la Piel.* Revista Mejicana de Dermatologia, 2008 (52) pag. 211-214. https://www.medigraphic.com/pdfs/derrevmex/rmd-2008/rmd085b.pdf

3.-Arrieta, Ana Santos. *Sistema GALT y traslocación Bacteriana.* Revista Heath & Medicine. Mayo 2016.

https://www.slideshare.net/anniesantos3139/galt-y-translocacion-bacteriana

4.-Serra, Jaume. *7 claves para potenciar el sistema inmunitario.* Revista Cuerpo Mente. Enero 2020 11:52.

https://www.cuerpomente.com/salud-natural/terapias-naturales/7-formar-potenciar-sistema-inmunitario_4255

5.-Puig, Ramiro E. *El Intestino : pieza clave del sistema inmunitario.* Revista Española de Enfermedades Digestivas. Volumen 100 # 1. Madrid Enero 2008. http://scielo.isciii.es/scielo.php?script=sci_arttext&pid=S1130-01082008000100006

6.-Shanahan F. The intestinal immune system. In: Johnson LR, editor. Physiology of the gastrointestinal tract. New York: Raven Press; 1994. p. 643-84.

7.-Smith DW, Nagler-Anderson C. Preventing intolerance : The induction of nonresponsiveness to dietary and microbial antigens in the intestinal mucosa. J Immunol 2005; 174: 3851-7.

8.-Woof JM, Mestecky J. Mucosal immunoglobuli. Immunol Rev 2005; 206: 64-82

Chapter 3

1. Rezaie A, Buresi M, Lembo A, et al. Hydrogen and methane based breath testing in gastrointestinal disorders: The North American Consensus. Am J gastroenterol 2017; 112: 775-84.

2. Calloway D, Calasito D, Mathew R. Gases produced by human intestinal flora. Nature. 1966; 212: 1238

3. Levitt M, Donald son R. Use of respiratory hydrogen (H2) excretion to detect carbohydrate malabsorption. J Lab Clin Med. 1970; 75: 937-45.

4. Ravich V, Bayless T, Thomas M. Fructose: incomplete intestinal absorption in humans. Gastroenterology. 1983; 84: 26

5. Domínguez-Jiménez J, Fernández A, Ruiz S, et al. Test de tolerancia a la lactosa reducido a 30 minutos: un estudio exploratorio de su facilidad e impacto. Rev Esp Enferm Dig. 2014; 106: 381-5

6. Yang J, DFox M, Chu H, et al. Four-sample lactose hydrogen breath test for diagnosis of lactose malabsorption in irritable bowel syndrome patients with diarrhea. Worl J Gastroenterol. 2015; 21: 7563-70.

7: 312-7. 17. Álvarez M, Miquel JF, Ibáñez P. Intolerancia a la lactosa. En: Enfermedades del colon e intestino. 2007.

8. Petschow B, Doré J, Hibberd P, et al. Probiots, prebiots and the host microbiome: The science of translation. Am N Y Acad Sci. 2013; 1306: 1-17.

9. Quigley E. and Quera R. Small intestinal bacterial overgrowth: Roles of antibiotics, prebiotics and probiotics. Gastroenterology. 2006; 30 (suppl 2): 578-90.

10. Sahakian A, Jees S, Pimentel M. Methane and gastrointestinal tract. Dig Dis Sci. 2010; 55: 2135-43.

11. Saad R, Chey W. Breath testing for small intestinal bacterial overgrowth. Maximizing test accurancy. Clin Gastroenterolo Hepatol. 2014; 12: 1964-72.

12.-Di Stefano M, Veneto G, Malservisi A, et al. Lactose malabsorption and intolerance in the elderly. Scand J Gastroenterol. 2001; 12: 1274–8.

13.-Van Rossum H, Van Rossum, Van Geenen E, et al. The one-hour lactose tolerance test. Clin Chem Lab Med. 2013; 51: 2

14.-Vonk R, Stellaard F, Priebe M, et al. The 13C/H2 glucose test for determination of small intestinal lactase activity. Eur J Clin Invest. 2001; 31: 226–33.

15.-Fell, P. Brostoff y M. Pasula. *Alta correlación entre los resultados del test de intolerancias alimentarias ALCAT y el desafío doble ciego en sensibilidades alimentarias*. Publicado en Annals of Allergy. 1988.

16.-Solomon, B. "*El ALCAT test : una guía y barómetro en la terapia para las Intolerancias Alimentarias y del Medioambiente. Environmental Medicine, vol. 9, 1992.*

Chapter 4

1.-Akcay, Mufide Nuren. *La Presencia de anticuerpos antigliadina en enfermedades tiroideas autoinmunes*. Revista de Hepatogastroenterologia Diciembre 2003, 50 Suppl. 2. https://pubmed.ncbi.nlm.nih.gov/15244201/

2.- Prevalencia y diagnóstico precoz de la enfermedad celíaca en trastornos tiroideos autoinmunes.[1] Cuoco L, Certo M, Jorizzo RA, De Vitis I, Tursi A, J Gastroenterol Hepatol. Mayo de 1999; 31 (4): 283-7.PMID: 10425571

3.- Conferencia de UCLA. Enfermedades tiroideas autoinmunes: de Graves y de Hashimoto.[2] Ann Intern Med. Mar de 1978; 88 (3): 379-91.PMID: 204241 Revisión.

4.-Guidetti, Sategna. *"Enfermedades tiroideas autoinmunes y enfermedad celiaca"*. Eus J Gastroenterol Hepatol. Noviembre 1998, 10 (11) : 927-31. https://pubmed.ncbi.nlm.nih.gov/9872614/

5.-Strieder, Thea. *Factores de riesgo y prevalencia de trastornos tiroideos en un estudio transversal entre mujeres sanas familiares de pacientes con enfermedad tiroidea autoinmune.* https://pubmed.ncbi.nlm.nih.gov/12919165/

6.-Hakanen, M. *Enfermedad tiroidea autoinmune clínica y subclínica en la enfermedad celíaca del* adulto. Dig Dis Sci Diciembre 2001. 46 (12) : 2631-51. https://pubmed.ncbi.nlm.nih.gov/11768252/

7.-Mainardi, Elsa. *Autoanticuerpos relacionados con la tiroides y enfermedad celíaca: ¿un papel para una dieta sin gluten?*. J Clin Gastroenterol. Sep 2002. 35 (3) 245-8. https://pubmed.ncbi.nlm.nih.gov/12192201/

8.- Diferencias en el consumo de alimentos entre pacientes con tiroiditis de Hashimoto e individuos sanos.[3] Kaličanin D, Brčić L, Ljubetić K, Barić A, Gračan S, Brekalo M, Torlak Lovrić V, Kolčić I, Polašek O, Zemunik T, Punda A, Boraska Perica V.Sci Rep.2020 30 de junio; 10 (1): 10670. doi: 10.1038 / s41598-020-67719-7.

9.- Marwaha RK, Garg MK, J. Glutamic acid decarboxylase (anti-GAD) & tissue transglutaminase (anti-TTG) antibodies in patients with thyroid autoimmunity.[4] Med Res. 2013 Jan;137(1):82-6. https://pubmed.ncbi.nlm.nih.gov/23481055/

10.- Metso S, Hyytiä-Ilmonen H, Kaukinen K. *Dieta sin gluten y tiroiditis autoinmune en pacientes celíacos. Un estudio prospectivo controlado.*[5] Scand J

---

1.   https://pubmed.ncbi.nlm.nih.gov/10425571/

2.   https://pubmed.ncbi.nlm.nih.gov/204241/

3.   https://pubmed.ncbi.nlm.nih.gov/32606353/

4.   https://pubmed.ncbi.nlm.nih.gov/23481055/

5.   *https://pubmed.ncbi.nlm.nih.gov/22126672/*

Gastroenterol. Enero de 2012; 47 (1): 43-8. https://pubmed.ncbi.nlm.nih.gov/12192201/

Chapter 5

1.-Rosen E, Materossian K, Grimm L. The role of vitamin D as a piece of the uterine factor infertility puzzle. Fertility and Sterility, 2019, 112(3): e35.

2.-Anagnostis P, Karras S, Goulis D. Vitamin D in human reproduction: a narrative review. Int J Clin Pract, March 2013, 67, 3, 225-235.

3.- Moreno, I., Codoñer, F. M., Vilella, F., Valbuena, (2016). Evidence that the endometrial microbiota has an effect on implantation success or failure. *American Journal of Obstetrics and Gynecology, 215(6),684703.*
https://doi.org/https://doi.org/10.1016/j.ajog.2016.09.075

4.- *Chinese herbal medicine for female infertility: an updated meta-analysis.*[1] Ried K.Complement Ther Med. 2015 Feb;23(1):116-28. doi: 10.1016/j.ctim.2014.12.004. Epub 2015 Jan 3.PMID: 25637159 Review.

5.- Influence of acupuncture on the pregnancy rate in patients who undergo assisted reproduction therapy. Paulus W et al, Fertil Steril 2002 Vol 77, pg 721-724

6.- Influence of acupuncture stimulation on pregnancy rates for women undergoing embryo transfer, Smith C et al, Fertil Steril 2006 Vol 85, pg 1352-1358

7.-Increase of success rate for women undergoing embryo transfer by transcutaneous electrical acupoint stimulation: a prospective randomized placebo-controlled study. Zhang R et al, Fertil Steril 2011, 96, 4 Pg 912-916,

8.-*Herbal Medicines and Ovarian Hyperstimulation Syndrome: A Retrospective Cohort Study.*[2] Rasekhjahromi A, Hosseinpoor M, Alipour F, Maalhagh M, Sobhanian S.Obstet Gynecol Int. 2016;2016:7635185. doi: 10.1155/2016/7635185. Epub 2016 Sep

9.-Fertility Madrid, Centro de Reproducción asistida : https://fertilitymadrid.com/blog-fertilidad/afecta-el-peso-a-la-fertilidad/

10.- Editor Zamora : https://vitaminad.mx/infertilidad-y-vitamina-d/

11.-https://www.reproduccionasistida.org/beneficios-de-la-acupuntura-para-la-fertilidad/ Dr. Juan C. Castillo, Enero 2019

---

1.   *https://pubmed.ncbi.nlm.nih.gov/25637159/*

2.   *https://pubmed.ncbi.nlm.nih.gov/27688772/*

Chapter 6

1.-Arranz R, Bendaña A, Bueno J, et al. Protocolo de Diagnóstico y Tratamiento de la Aplasia Medular. Asociación Española de Hematología y Hemoterapia, Subcomité de Aplasia Medular del Grupo Español de Trasplante de Progenitores Hematopoyéticos 2001: 1-12. http://www.carloshaya.net/uchematologia/media/aplasia.pdf.

2.- Bacigalupo A, Passweg J. Diagnosis and Treatment of Acquired Aplastic Anemia. Hematol Oncol Clin N Am 2009; 23: 159–170

3.- Malik S, Sarwar I, Mehmood T, Naz F. Etiological Considerations of Acquired Aplastic Anemia. J Ayub Med Coll Abbottabad 2009; 21(3): 127-13.

4.- http://whsc.emory.edu/soundscience/archives/lonial.html Woodruff Health Science Center. Cuando la Médula ósea se estropea. Sagar Lonial, MD.

5.- El rol de las vitaminas en la prevención y el control de la anemia.

6.-Steel K, Gertman PM, Crescenzi C, Anderson J. (1981). Iatrogenic illness on a general medical service at a university hospital. N Engl J Med. 304:638-42.

7.-https://web.archive.org/web/20101218033809/ http://fihu-diagnostico.org.pe/revista/numeros/2004/oct-dic04/229-232.html. Albújar P. Iatrogenia. Diagnóstico. 2044; 43(5).[1]

8.- Leape L.Unecessarsary surgery. Annu Rev Public Health. 1992;13:363-383.

9.- Phillips D, Christenfeld N, Glynn L. Increase in US medication-error deaths between 1983 and 1993. Lancet. 1998;351:643

10.- Lazarou J, Pomeranz B, Corey P. Incidence of adverse drug reactions in hospitalized patients. JAMA. 1998;279:1200-1205.

11.-Starfield, Bárbara, MD., "Los Médicos son la tercera causa de muerte en los Estados Unidos". Escuela de Higiene y Salud Pública John Hopkins. Journal of the American Medical Association (JAMA), 1999.

1.	https://web.archive.org/web/20101218033809/http:/fihu-diagnostico.org.pe/revista/numeros/2004/oct-dic04/229-232.html

Chapter 7

1.-https://www.clinicafuensalud.com/paralisis-facial-tratada-con-acupuntura/. *"parálisis facial tratada con acupuntura*. Febrero 2020.

2.- https://www.salud180.com/salud-dia-dia/combate-vitamina-b6-paralisis-facial

3.-https://www.doctoralia.com.mx/preguntas-respuestas/el-complejo-b-sirve-para-prevenir-la-paralisis-facial

4.-*https://espanol.ninds.nih.gov/trastornos/paralisis_de_bell.htm Parálisis de Bell. National Institute of Neurological Disorders and Stroke (NIH).*

5.-Clínica Mayo, información al paciente y educación médica. https://www.mayoclinic.org/es-es/diseases-conditions/bells-palsy/symptoms-causes/syc-20370028

6.- https://www.murciasalud.es/preevid/15555. De los tratamientos empleados en la parálisis facial periférica idiopática,¿cuáles han demostrado su eficacia?.

7.-Zandian A, Osiro S, *et al.* The neurologist's dilemma. A comprehensive clinical review of Bell's palsy, with emphasis on current management trends. Med Sc Monit. 2014; 20: 83-90. Disponible en: http://www.ncbi.nlm.nih.gov/pmc/articles/PMC3907546/

8.-Xia F, Han J, Liu X, Wang J, Jiang Z, Wang K, *et al.* Prednisolone and acupuncture in Bell's palsy: study protocol for a randomized, controlled trial. Trial. 2011 [citado 20 dic 2014]; 12: 158. Disponible en: http://www.ncbi.nlm.nih.gov/pubmed/21693007

9.-He X, Zhu Y, *et al.* Acupuncture-induced changes in functional connectivity of the primary somatosensory cortex varied with pathological stages of Bell's palsy. Neuroreport. 2014; 25(14): 1162-8. http://www.ncbi.nlm.nih.gov/pubmed/25121624

10.-Díaz Barrios H. Efectividad del tratamiento acupuntural en la parálisis facial periférica. (Tesis). Pinar del Río: Hospital clínico quirúrgico docente Abel Santamaría; 2002.

Chapter 8

1.-AskMayoExpert. Colorectal cancer: Screening and management (adult). Rochester, Minn.: Mayo Foundation for Medical Education and Research; 2018.

2.-Colon cancer. Plymouth Meeting, Pa.: National Comprehensive Cancer Network. https://www.nccn.org/professionals/physician_gls/default.aspx. Accessed Jan., 2019.

3.-Macrae FA. Colorectal cancer: Epidemiology, risk factors and protective factors. https://www.uptodate.com/contents/search. Accessed Feb. 5, 2019

4.-Grothey A, et al. Duration of adjuvant chemotherapy for stage III colon cancer. New England Journal of Medicine. 2018;378:1177.

5.-https://www.cancer.org/es/tratamiento/supervivencia-durante-y-despues-del-tratamiento/bienestar-durante-el-tratamiento/nutricion.html

6.- Naidu KA: Vitamin C in human health and disease is still a mystery? An overview. Nutr J 2: 7, 2003. [PUBMED Abstract][1]

7.- Cameron E, Pauling L: The orthomolecular treatment of cancer. I. The role of ascorbic acid in host resistance. Chem Biol Interact 9 (4): 273-83, 1974. [PUBMED Abstract][2]

8.-Cameron E, Campbell A: The orthomolecular treatment of cancer. II. Clinical trial of high-dose ascorbic acid supplements in advanced human cancer. Chem Biol Interact 9 (4): 285-315, 1974. [PUBMED Abstract][3]

9.- Cameron E, Pauling L: Supplemental ascorbate in the supportive treatment of cancer: Prolongation of survival times in terminal human cancer. Proc Natl Acad Sci U S A 73 (10): 3685-9, 1976. [PUBMED Abstract][4]

10.- Moertel CG, Fleming TR, Creagan ET, et al.: High-dose vitamin C versus placebo in the treatment of patients with advanced cancer who have had no prior chemotherapy. A randomized double-blind comparison. N Engl J Med 312 (3): 137-41, 1985. [PUBMED Abstract][5]

---

1.   http://www.ncbi.nlm.nih.gov/entrez/
query.fcgi?cmd=Retrieve&db=PubMed&list_uids=14498993&dopt=Abstract

2.   http://www.ncbi.nlm.nih.gov/entrez/
query.fcgi?cmd=Retrieve&db=PubMed&list_uids=4609626&dopt=Abstract

3.   http://www.ncbi.nlm.nih.gov/entrez/
query.fcgi?cmd=Retrieve&db=PubMed&list_uids=4430016&dopt=Abstract

4.   http://www.ncbi.nlm.nih.gov/entrez/
query.fcgi?cmd=Retrieve&db=PubMed&list_uids=1068480&dopt=Abstract

5.   http://www.ncbi.nlm.nih.gov/entrez/
query.fcgi?cmd=Retrieve&db=PubMed&list_uids=3880867&dopt=Abstract

Chapter 9

1.-Becker, Simon A. Un Ritalin Alternativo. Acupuntura en el tratamiento del TDAH. Psiquiatría Médica China. Amapola azul Empresas: 2007.

2.-Hong, Harry. El tratamiento de los niños con TDAH de forma natural. HealthBoards: Consultado el 5 de junio de 2007. & lt; http://www.healthboards.com/boards/archive/index.php/t-8818.html& Gt;

3.-Acupuntura para tratar el déficit de atención con o sin hiperactividad (TDAH y TDA). https://acupunturainfo.com/tdah/

4.-Abikoff, H.B., Thompson, M., Laver-Bradbury, C., Long, N., Forehand, R. L., Miller Brotman, L., et al. (2015). Parent training for preschool ADHD: a randomized controlled trial of specialized and generic programs. *Journal of Child Psychology and Psychiatry, 56*, 618-31.

5.-Barbaresi, W. J., Colligan, R. C., Weaver, A. L., Voigt, R. G., Killian, J. M., & Katusic, S. K. (2013). Mortality, ADHD, and psychosocial adversity in adults with childhood ADHD: a prospective study. *Pediatrics, 131*(4), 637-644.

6.- Libro de Clínica Mayo, *"Guía para criar a un niño saludable". https://www.mayoclinic.org/es-es/diseases-conditions/adhd/symptoms-causes/ syc-20350889*

7.- David Wolfe, Dieta para el TDAH : 5 alimentos que debe evitar. https://www.conocersalud.com/dieta-tdah/

Chapter 10

1.-Muchachas anoréxicas y bulímicas de Mateo Selvini Palazzoli, Mara Selvini Palazzoli, Sthefano Cirilo y A.M. Sorrentino. Editorial Paidos. 1999.

2.-Las prisiones de la comida de Giorgio Nardone, Roberta Milanese y Tiziana Verbitz, Editorial Herder. 2002..

3.-American Psychiatric Association. Practice guidelines for the treatment of patients with eating disorders, third edition. Am J Psychiatry 2006; 163(Suppl): 1-50

4.-Asociación Americana de Psiquiatría. (2014). Manual diagnóstico y estadístico de los trastornos mentales (DSM-5). 5ª Ed. Arlington, VA, Asociación Americana de Psiquiatría: Panamericana.

5.-Barrera, A. (2016). Impulsividad y TDAH en pacientes adolescentes con trastornos de conducta alimentaria. Tesis doctoral. Enlace[1].

6.-Bleichmar, H. (2014). La Anorexia. En "Curso de especialista en clínica y psicoterapia psicoanalítica". Madrid.

7.-Doyen, C. y Cook-Darzens, S. (2005). Anorexia, Bulimia: pautas para prevenir, afrontar y actuar desde la infancia. 1º edición. Barcelona: Amat.

8.-Madruga, A. D., Leis, T. R. & Lambruschini, F. N. (2010). Trastornos del comportamiento alimentario: Anorexia nerviosa y bulimia nerviosa. En: Asociación Española de Pediatria.

---

1.   https://zaguan.unizar.es/record/56685/files/TESIS-2016-183.pdf

Chapter 11

1.- Stevens DA, Kan VL, Judson MA, et al. Practice guidelines for diseases caused by *Aspergillus, Clin Infect Dis, 2000, vol 30*pg. 696-70).

3.-Marr KA, Patterson T, Denning D. Aspergillosis: pathogenesis, clinical manifestations, and therapy. *Infect Dis Clin North Am.* 2002, vol 16 (pag. 875-94.

4.- Walsh TJ, Petraitiene V, et al. Experimental pulmonary aspergillosis due to *Aspergillus terreus:* pathogenesis and treatment of an emerging fungal pathogen resistant to amphotericin B. J Infect Dis, 2003, vol 188 (pag. 305-19).

5.- Willems L, van der Geest R, de Beule K. Itraconazole oral solution and intravenous formulations: a review of pharmacokinetics and pharmacodynamics. *J Clin Pharm Ther, 2001, vol 26, pag. 159-69*

6.-Nair, M. K. M., J. Joy, et al. (2005). "Antibacterial Effect of Caprylic Acid and Monocaprylin on Major Bacterial Mastitis Pathogens." Journal of dairy science 88(10): 3488-3495.

7.- Wang J, Huang N, Xiong J, Wei H, Jiang S, Peng J. Caprylic acid and nonanoic acid upregulate endogenous host defense peptides to enhance intestinal epithelial immunological barrier function via histone deacetylase inhibition[1]. Int Immunopharmacol. 2018 Oct 17;65:303-311. doi: 10.1016/j.intimp.2018.10.022.

8.-Li Y. The application of caprylic acid in downstream processing of monoclonal antibodies[2]. Protein Expr Purif. 2019 Jan;153:92-96. doi: 10.1016/j.pep.2018.09.003. Epub 2018 Sep 8.

9.-Kim HW, Rhee MS. Response surface modeling of reductions in uropathogenic Escherichia coli biofilms on silicone by cranberry extract, caprylic acid, and thymol[3]. Biofouling. 2018 Sep 6:1-8. doi: 10.1080/08927014.2018.1488969.

10.-https://alergiaalpolen.com/es-buena-la-leche-para-el-asma-la-alergia/. indalocodex@gmail.com . Leche, asma y alergias. Xaverio 2020.

---

1.   https://www.ncbi.nlm.nih.gov/pubmed/30342347

2.   https://www.ncbi.nlm.nih.gov/pubmed/30205153

3.   https://www.ncbi.nlm.nih.gov/pubmed/30187778

Chapter 12

1.-Puig, Ramiro E. *El Intestino : pieza clave del sistema inmunitario.* Revista Española de Enfermedades Digestivas. Volumen 100 # 1. Madrid Enero 2008. http://scielo.isciii.es/ scielo.php?script=sci_arttext&pid=S1130-01082008000100006

2.-Mowat AM. Anatomical basis of tolerance and immunity to intestinal antigens. Nat Rev Immunol 2003; 3: 331-41.

3.- Smith DW, Nagler-Anderson C. Preventing intolerance: The induction of nonresponsiveness to dietary and microbial antigens in the intestinal mucosa. J Immunol 2005; 174: 3851-7.

4.- Chambers SJ, Wickham MS, Regoli M, Bertelli E, Gunning PA, Nicoletti C. Rapid in vivo transport of proteins from digested allergen across pre-sensitized gut. Biochem Biophys Res Commun 2004; 325: 1258-63.

5.-Alergia e intolerancia alimentaria en la Artritis Reumatoidea. Blog informativo sobre la Artritis Reumatoidea del Centro Médico de Enfermedades Reumáticas "Artricenter". https://artritisreumatoid.wordpress.com/2014/12/04/alergia-e-intolerancia-alimentaria-en-la-artritis-reumatoide/

6.-Los Niños y la Artritis. Una guía para salir adelante. Boletín para pacientes 4. Asociación Peruana de Reumatología. 1996.

7.- Berrocal A, Ferrándiz M y Calvo A. Metotrexate en Artritis Reumatoide juvenil. Informe Preliminar. Medicina Moderna. 1993; 1: 3-6.

8.-Tratamientos efectivos para la Artritis totalmente naturales. https://www.bloglines.com/article/effective-all-natural-arthritis-treatments?ad=dirN&qo=serpIndex&o=740010

9.- Lactose Intolerance in Adults: Biological Mechanism and Dietary Management. Yanyong Deng, Benjamin Misselwitz, Ning Dai, Mark Fox. Nutrients 2015, 7, 8020-8035. https://www.ncbi.nlm.nih.gov/pmc/articles/PMC4586575/.

10.-Hipersensibilidad Alimentaria. Medicina Interna Basada en Evidencias, Manual MIBE. https://empendium.com/manualmibe/chapter/B34.II.4.26.

Chapter 13

1.-Bordelon P, Ghetu MV, Langan RC. Reconocimiento y manejo de la deficiencia de vitamina D . *Soy Fam Physician* . 2009; 80 (8): 841–846

2.-Tangpricha V. et all. Deficiencia de vitamina D y trastornos relacionados. http://emedicine.medscape.com/article/128762-overview . Consultado el 4 de noviembre de 2014.

3.-Melville NA. USPSTF : no hay evidencia de pruebas de detección de vitamina D de rutina. Consultado el 3/12/2014.http://www.medscape.com/viewarticle/835369 .

4.-Nogales-Gaete J, Jiménez P, García P, Sáez D, Aracena R, González et al. Mielopatía por déficit de vitamina B 12: caracterización clínica de 11 casos. *Rev Méd Chile* 2004; 132: 1377-82.

5.-Aaron S, Kumar S, Vijayan J, Jacob J, Alexander M, Gnanamuthu C. Clinical and laboratory features and response to treatment in patients presenting with vitamin B12 deficiency-related neurological syndromes. *Neurol India* 2005; 53: 55-8; discussion 59.

6.-Lumbalgias y lumbociatalgias tratadas mediante electroacupuntura. Rev Int Acupuntura 2008. Discussions on real-world acupuncture treatments for chronic low-back pain in older adults. Journal of Integrative Medicine 2019.

7.- Collazo E. Efectividad de la acupuntura en el alivio del dolor refractario al tratamiento farmacológico convencional. Rev Soc Esp Dolor. 2009; 16(2): 79-86.

8.- Gonzáles S, Rodrígus R, Caballero A, Selva A. Eficacia Terapéutica de la acupuntura en pacientes con sacrolumbalgia. MEDISAN. 2011; 15(3). 1029-3019

Chapter 14

1.-Akera T: Pharmacological agents and myocardial calcium, in Langer GA (ed): Calcium and the Heart. New York, Raven Press Ltd, 1990, p 299. 2.

2.- Nelson MT, Patlak JB, Worley JF, Standen NB. Calcium channels, potassium channels and voltage dependence of arterial smooth muscle tone. Am J Physiol Cell Physiol 1990; 259: C3-C18. 10.

3.- Lancet, 338; pg. 667; 14 Sep 1991. Magnesio y corazón

4.- Whelton, P.K. y Klag, M.J. Am.J.Cardiol., 63; pg. 26G-30G; 1989. Magnesio y salud cardiovascular

5.- Resnick, L.M. Proc.Nat.Acad.Sc. (USA), 81; pg.6511-15; 1984. Magnesio y Arritmias.

6.- Dycner, T. y Wester, P.O.. Br.Med.J., 286; pg.1847-9; 1983. Magnesio y ritmo cardíaco

7.- Dycner, T. y Wester, P.O. Lacnet, 1; pg.585-6; 1981. Magnesio como antiarrítmico

8.-*Ernster L,(1995). "Aspectos bioquímicos, fisiológicos y médicos de la función de ubiquinona". Biochimica et Biophysica Acta- Bases moleculares de la enfermedad . 1271 (1): 195-204.*

9.-*Flowers N, Hartley L, Todkill D, Stranges S, Rees K (4 de diciembre de 2014). "Suplementación de coenzima Q10 para la prevención primaria de enfermedades cardiovasculares". La* base de datos Cochrane de revisiones sistemáticas . 12 (12): CD010405.

10.-Cardioprotective effect of L-Carnitine in rats submitted to permanent left coronary artery ligation. Arch Intern Physiol Biochim Biophys 1993; 101: 411-416.

11.-Effects of L-Carnitine on ventricular arrithmias after coronary reperfusion. Jpn Circ J 1983; 47: 536-542.

Don't miss out!

Visit the website below and you can sign up to receive emails whenever Sergio A. Chacón M. publishes a new book. There's no charge and no obligation.

https://books2read.com/r/B-A-EFTAB-LONQC

BOOKS 2 READ

Connecting independent readers to independent writers.